Frontier Military Series
XX

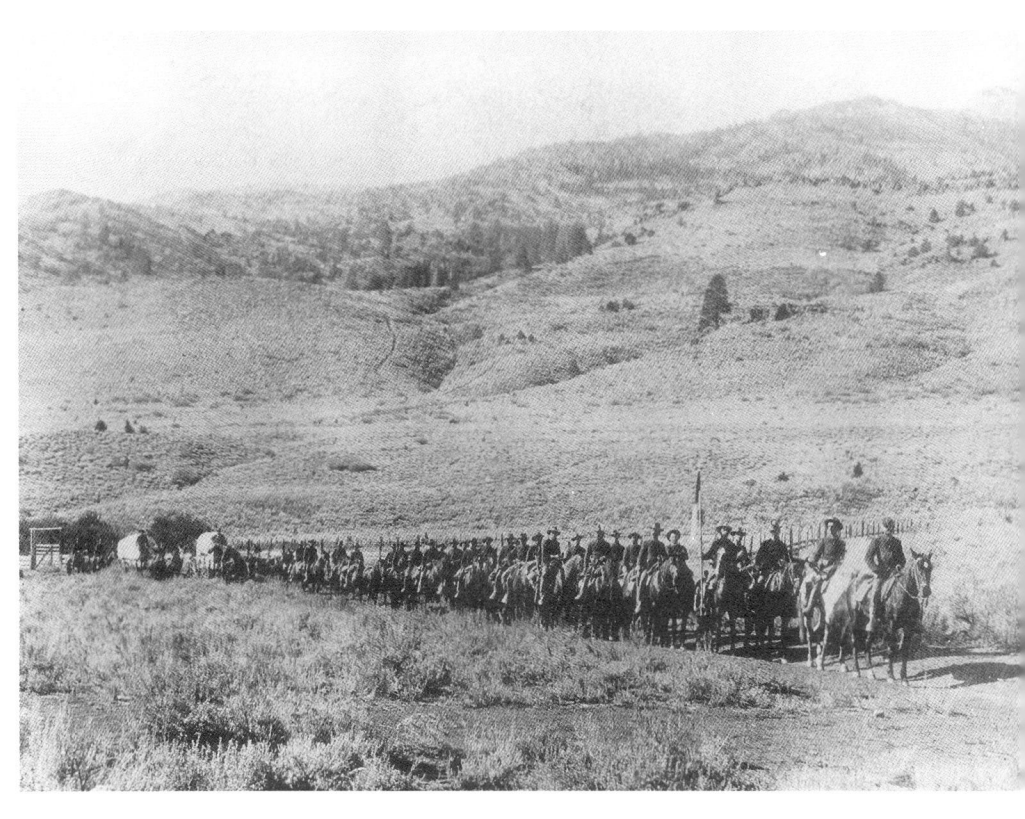

Troops departing Fort Bidwell for the last time, 1893.
Courtesy, Patricia A. Berry

A SAW,
POCKET INSTRUMENTS,
and
TWO OUNCES OF WHISKEY

Frontier Military Medicine
in the Great Basin

by
Anton Paul Sohn

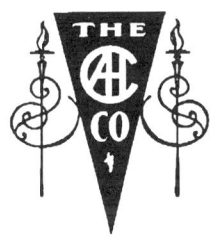

THE ARTHUR H. CLARK COMPANY
Spokane, Washington
1998

Arthur H. Clark Company
P.O. Box 14707
Spokane, WA 99214

LIBRARY OF CONGRESS CATALOG CARD NUMBER 96-30690
ISBN-0-87062-272-2

Library of Congress Cataloging-in-Publication Data

Sohn, A. P. (Anton Paul), 1935—
    A saw, pocket instruments, and two ounces of whiskey: frontier
military medicine in the Great Basin / by Anton Paul Sohn.
        p. 240   cm.— (Frontier military series ; 20)
    Includes bibliographical references and index.
    ISBN 0-87062-272-2 (alk. paper)
1. Medicine, Military —Great Basin—History—19th century.
I. Title.   II. Series.
RC971.S627   1998   97-30690
616.9'8023'097909034—dc21   CIP

Contents

Illustrations

Preface

A goal of the History of Medicine Program at the University of Nevada School of Medicine is to research the history of medicine in Nevada. When the program began in 1987, I hoped to provide the stimulus for someone to undertake this project. The idea gestated for five years in my mind before I decided to write the story of the first doctors—the military surgeons—in all of the Great Basin, not just the State of Nevada. I hope the accumulation of this effort will illuminate events in this region and provide an understanding of the medical sciences and military medicine in the nineteenth century. The material in this book is the first chapter of the medical history of a unique region in the United States.

In many ways the story is not unique. The Army, protecting the citizens and inhabitants, provided the first physicians to the region as it did in many parts of the country. The Civil War momentarily interrupted their efforts and the settlement of the West, but it also brought about new methods and innovations of caring for the sick and wounded. Furthermore, medical discoveries, including the bacterial cause of disease, in the last quarter of the nineteenth century, changed the face of medical science and the prevalence of the many diseases chronicled in this saga. For instance, malaria, a devastating disease during the early days on the Great Basin frontier, would become a curiosity.

The story in this book took place during the second half of the nineteenth century. Unfortunately, some records have been destroyed by fire and others lost, but the remaining records tell a story of adventure, life, death, and just as important, a devotion to humanity. I encourage those who wish to pursue the subject further to search for information on the actors in this drama who are only names in an appendix.

My indebtedness to those who helped make this work possible is beyond calculation. I am deeply indebted to Professor emeritus and Physician Robert J. T. Joy at the Uniformed Services University of the Health Sciences for his wise counsel, editorial suggestions, and knowledge of military medicine and history. A better choice to write the Foreword for this book could not have been made. I was somewhat reluctant to ask Dr. Joy to lend his approval to this work because he is the leading authority in the country on the subject and far more knowledgeable than I. Fortunately, he agreed.

I am particularly grateful to Guy Louis Rocha, the Nevada State Archivist, who provided a historical perspective of Nevada, and Patricia A. Barry of Fort Bidwell who shared her photographs and information on Fort Bidwell and George Martin Kober, but also lent a keen, English teacher's eye to a pathologist. Furthermore, I am indebted to Edward T. Morman, former Medical History Librarian at Johns Hopkins University, and now at the New York Academy of Medicine and Diana L. McAninch, former Managing Editor of the Western Journal of Medicine, who read the manuscript and offered criticism and suggestions.

Much of my research on the military physicians in the Great Basin took place at the National Archives in Washington, D. C., and would not have been possible without the help of Historian Michael P. Musick of the Military Reference Branch. His associate, Michael T. Meier, also of the Military Reference Branch, provided valuable information, and Mrs. Ruth Langham Gleason researched many of the early surgeon's personnel records.

Martina Ellis of Amite, Louisiana, kindly lent a copy of the Corbusier Journal. Charles G. Hibbard of the Fort Douglas Military Museum, provided valuable information and photographs pertinent to the medical history of Fort Douglas. Maggie Lowther, Storey County Recorder in Virginia City, provided a copy of Edmund Gardner Bryant's letter. Rodney Burow, Physician's Assistant at Fort McDermitt, provided photographs and information. Susan Miller Kerns graciously allowed me to locate the stone foundation of the Fort Scott hospital on her property. Dr. Owen C. Bolstad and Roy Hogan helped to survey the various forts and locate the hospitals. Dr. Thomas K. Hood, Sheldon Homer, Paul Sawyer, and Richard Immenschuh of Elko, Nevada, were instrumental in obtaining permission to locate the footings of Fort Halleck's hospitals and identifying the two remaining buildings at Fort Ruby.

The kindness and cooperation of the staffs of libraries, historical societies, medical societies, and museums in which research was undertaken or information provided is gratefully acknowledged. These include: Robert Boyd of The High Desert Museum, Bend, Oregon; William Michaels of the Eastern California Museum in Independence, California; Phillip I. Earl of the Nevada Historical Society; Robert Nylen of the Nevada Museum; Jeffrey M. Kintop and George T. Earnhart of the Nevada State Library and Archives; Ulla Lipp and Nancy Masters of the Inyo County Library in Independence, California; Jami Frazier Tracy of the Wichita-Sedgwick County Historical Museum in Kansas; Susan Ward of the Kansas Medical Society; Sharon Allen and J. P. Marden of the Humboldt County Library in Winnemucca; Sharon M. Jones of the Harney County Historical Museum in Oregon; Tom McMasters of the United States Army Medical Department Museum; and librarians at the National Library of Medicine, Library of Congress, California State Library, Bancroft Library in Berkeley, Lane Medical Library at Stanford University, University of California Special Collections in San Francisco, Northeastern Nevada Museum, University of Nevada, Reno Special Collections Department, Society of California Pioneers, and University of Nevada School of Medicine. Others I consider crucial in preparation of this manuscript are Nita R. Spangler of Redwood City, California; Carolyn Beaupre of Virginia City, Nevada; Tanya Leonesio of Reno; Edna Patterson of Elko, Nevada; James Prida, Fort Churchill Park Supervisor; Gary N. Tjader of Los Altos, California; and Linda Duferrena of Winnemucca. I am also indebted to Eileen Barker and Karen Cavallaro in the Department of Pathology at the University of Nevada School of Medicine for editing, suggestions, and assistance. My son, Anton Phillip Sohn, helped with computer formatting and my daughter, Kristin Diane Sohn, edited parts of the manuscript. Most important of all has been the aid and support given by my wife, Arlene Ann Sohn.

ANTON P. SOHN
University of Nevada
School of Medicine

FOREWORD
The Uses of Local History

Thomas Carlyle said in 1830 that "history is the essence of innumerable biographies;" eleven years later Emerson wrote that "there is properly no history, only biography." I offer a broader definition with a paraphrase of former House Speaker O'Neill's description of politics; I suggest that all history is local. No matter how deep the analysis, how synoptic the coverage, how broad the use of sources or how devoted to the current fads, historical writing will ultimately be based on studies of a locale and its people. Whether it is the history of a court, a battle, a social movement, a political event—the data will be assembled from local studies which may then be synthesized into larger and more sweeping narratives.

This careful description of the medical officers and contract physicians, their army posts, their medical practice and their patients' problems is local history at its best. Dr. Sohn prepared himself for this work with a sabbatical year at the Johns Hopkins Institute for the History of Medicine, and has founded a Great Basin medical history newsletter, a medical history course at the his medical school and an oral history program (and a publishing program for it).

The author's use of primary sources is impressive. The National Archives have been exploited in detail, oral history is used where possible, and previously unknown material such as letters and the Corbusier diary is well mined. Site visits and archeological explorations have been done wherever a surviving post and its hospital can be found. Secondary sources have been carefully consulted. In short, all the tools of historiography have been brought to bear to tell the story of military medicine in support of those soldiers in blue sent out to defend and expand the border marches of the nation.

To those who have attended to this aspect of military medical history in this era it is again demonstrated that disease, not battle, was the major cause of morbidity and mortality. It is important to note, as does the author, the similarities and differences between military and civilian medical problems. The Fort Churchill and Saint Mary Louise Hospital data illuminate this issue very nicely.

This book will be a very useful source for historians of old army posts, like the Council on American's Military Past, for curators of western museums and historians of the West and the United States Army in general. General readers interested in the history of "John Wayne's Army" will find here insights and information about the Great Basin available nowhere else. This book is the very model of what excellent local history should be; that it is so clearly and so well written is a bonus for the reader.

ROBERT J.T. JOY, MD, FACP
COL, MC, USA (Ret.)
Professor Emeritus, Medical History
Uniformed Services University of
    the Health SciencesBethesda, Md.

Frontier Military Medicine
on the Great Basin

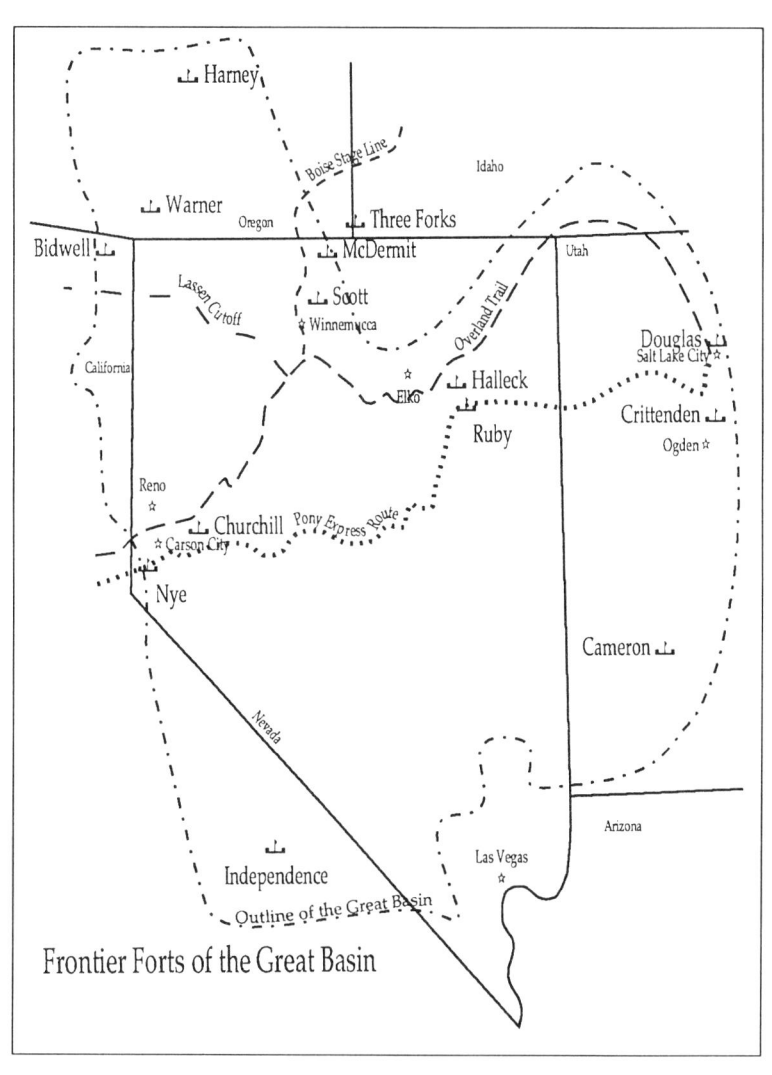

Frontier Forts of the Great Basin

Map prepared by the author and Anton Phillip Sohn

Prelude to the Military Physicians
on the Great Basin
1840-1857

For thirty-six years, from 1857-1893, the Great Basin[1] was the site of United States Army posts established to secure the frontier.[2] This land of arid desolate deserts, fertile valleys, rimrock bounded plateaus, high boxed canyons, and endless mountains is located between the steep Sierra Nevada of California on the west and the soaring Rocky Mountains on the east. The Great Basin comprises most of Nevada; adjacent areas of California, Oregon, and Utah; and a small area of southern Idaho.[3] During this thirty-six-year period on the western frontier, army hospitals provided health care for soldiers, and in fact, for all who needed assistance.

The military posts, originally intended to keep peace

---

[1]The name, Great Basin, was coined by John C. Fremont when he explored the region.

[2]A word of caution is necessary about the use of fort, post, camp, or other names to identify a military establishment. Although a fort has a connotation of a more permanent establishment, there was no rule as to the proper name to be used. It was usually derived from the order creating the base. Several Great Basin posts were established as camps and then later changed to forts. I use these terms loosely and make no attempt to determine when an official order changed a designation.

When Fort Bidwell closed in 1893, Fort Douglas in Utah was the only fort to exist beyond the frontier period as defined by the other military forts of the Great Basin. Coincidentally, 1893 is also the date that historian Frederick Jackson Turner, based on population densities drawn from the 1890 census, declared the frontier closed.

[3]This definition of the Great Basin is open to some controversy because the area can be defined by either its geology or hydrology.

between the Native Americans and non-native inhabitants and to prevent secession activity, provided organized medical care with trained physicians and hospitals. This, the Intermountain West, a land of extremes in terrain, elevation, and climate, and the last great frontier in the continental United States to be explored and settled, was a microcosm of health care in the United States. This discussion of the military medical doctors, their patients—soldiers and the inhabitants of the Great Basin—and the diseases they treated, focuses on nineteenth-century medicine and health hazards in the territory.

These military doctors, who are mostly faceless names, came from exceedingly varied backgrounds and circumstances. They were from many countries and like their civilian colleagues from many different educational backgrounds. A few had not graduated from medical school, but as a whole they were better educated than their civilian counterparts.[4] Some were commissioned officers in the army—a difficult position to obtain; others were civilians on contract; and some were Civil War volunteers.

Before military surgeons came to practice medicine in the Great Basin, Bannock, Paiute, Shoshone, Kawaiisu, Ute and Washoe healers had practiced their craft there for thousands of years. These Native Americans were truly the first doctors on the Great Basin desert. They also accompanied war and hunting parties for religious purposes.

The first non-native doctors encountered by the Indians were those intrepid American physicians accompanying the exploratory expeditions and wagon trains across the country to the West Coast in the 1840s. These wagon trains coursed the uncharted deserts of the Great Basin carrying emigrants and their belongings to California and Oregon. Between

---

[4]As will be discussed later, military doctors were carefully investigated before they were commissioned. On the other hand, there was no regulatory organization for civilian physicians.

1841, when the first overland wagon train reached California, and the Civil War, over 250,000 people traveled to the Pacific Coast through the Great Basin, and many didn't finish the trip and were buried along the trails.

The health care needs of such a large mass of humanity on the move taxed the accompanying physicians and sometimes impeded their own trip west while they stopped to treat sick and injured travelers. Many challenges faced the doctor on the trail. For example cholera, present in settlements across the country, became epidemic and spread among the emigrants trekking west. Dr. George W. Davis estimated that he treated over three hundred cases of cholera during his overland trip in 1850. Another physician calculated that he saw over seven hundred cases, while a third treated up to forty patients a day on the trail.[5]

Cholera killed many on the trails, but just as devastating was inadequately treated trauma or a complication during delivery of a newborn infant. A diary account described an all too often problem: infection from trauma and lack of competent medical treatment. A young boy had a leg crushed by a wagon wheel resulting in gangrene and maggots crawling in the wound. Unable to locate a doctor, his mother found a former medical student who rode twenty miles to help. A former surgeon's assistant, present in the company, "assembled a butcher knife, a carpenter's handsaw, and a shoemaker's awl to take up the arteries." The child was given laudanum, tied down, and "mercifully" died during the one hour and three quarters operation.[6]

Some of the civilian physicians traveling west nailed signs on their wagons and saw patients along the trails. Some even

---

[5]John D. Unruh, *The Plains Across: The Overland Emigrants and the Trans-Mississippi West, 1840-60*, p. 101. Sources found in the notes of this work are cited in full in the Bibiography.

[6]George R. Stewart, *The California Trail*, p. 154.

erra

them out for medical care. On occasion, travelers camped near a physician to have health care available. In contrast, there are records of physicians who traveled as far as eighty miles along the trails to see a patient.

To assure the services of a physician, many organized wagon trains paid doctors to accompany them on the long journey west. Those trained in New York City were the most sought after by the emigrants, but any available doctor would do. On one occasion a party of fifty, already half way through the overland trip, contracted with a doctor for $250.00 ($5 a person) to remain with the group for the remainder of the trip. Others were penniless and were treated *gratis*.[7] However, many emigrants were not so fortunate to find a doctor on the trail and made do with any remedy available.

In 1857 the army established its first post in the Great Basin at Camp Floyd near Salt Lake City. For the first time, army doctors were available for emergencies and medical care in the territory. As was the case in many areas of the country, these military surgeons were the first organized group of doctors devoted to the full-time practice of medicine.[8] The Army also built the first hospitals, located on military reservations, that served soldiers as well as civilians.

Records from many of the military posts listed hospitalized civilian patients. Only rarely were Native Americans admitted to a military hospital. Assistant Surgeon Washington Matthews at Fort Independence indicated in May 1876 that there were three patients on the sick roll including "our one and only Indian Scout, [Joe Bowers] so nicknamed." He suffered from pains and abscesses, "apparently of syphilic ori-

---

[7]Unruh, *The Plains Across*, pp. 97, 101.

[8]The first attempt to establish the Nevada State Medical Association was made July 1, 1878. Twenty-four doctors attended and 33 were on the membership roll. The first president was Dr. J. W. Van Zandt. See Angel, ed., *History of Nevada;* Poulson, Helen J., *Index to Thompson and West's History of Nevada,* Bibliographical Series, No. 6, p. 261-62. The Utah State Medical Association was organized in 1897. In 1904 the Nev. State Med. Assoc. was re-established.

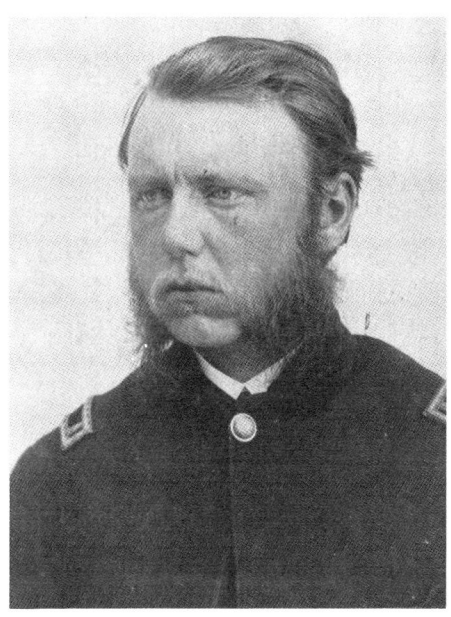

Army Doctor
Washington Mathews
Courtesy of National Library
of Medicine

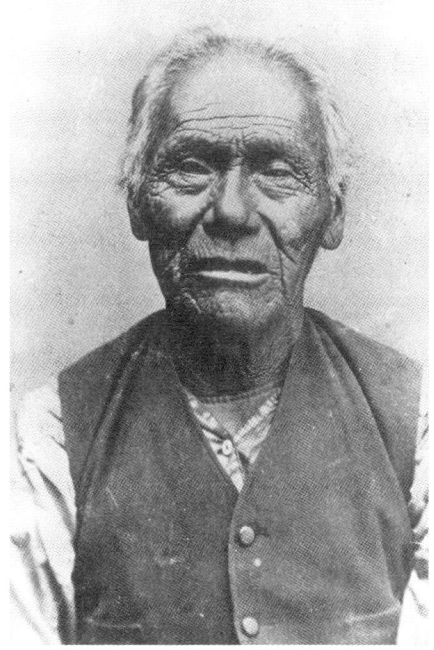

Indian Scout Joe Bowers
Courtesy of Eastern California
Museum

suffered from pains and abscesses, "apparently of syphilic origin." According to records, he was lonely for his friends and
home in the White Mountains. He left the hospital against
Matthew's advice.⁹ Another Native American with a frac-
tured fibula was segregated in an outbuilding as a charity
patient at Fort Independence.[10]

There were many instances where Indians living near or at
Great Basin forts received medical care from the post surgeon. In fact, on occasion Indians served in the Army and
received medical care from the post doctor. The most notable
occasion occurred at Fort Douglas at the end of the nineteenth century. On February 3, 1892, Company "I," 16th
Infantry, comprised of fifty-five Sioux soldiers arrived at Fort
Douglas from the Rosebud Agency. When the company
departed May 28, 1894, there were only twenty-seven
remaining. Most of the missing twenty-eight had died as the
result of unspecified illness and one man had committed suicide after receiving the news of his father's death.[11]

After Fort Bidwell closed in 1893, Fort Douglas was the
last military base in the Great Basin. Army doctors were no
longer necessary for civilian or Native American health care.
By then medical service was well established in the major
population areas. However, prior to the military presence,
there were few, if any full-time practicing physicians in the
territory. There were physicians in the Mormon communities of Salt Lake City and Mormon Station (now Genoa,
Nevada), but it does not appear they practiced full-time.[12] In
fact, the few well-trained Mormon physicians were discour-

---

⁹Bowers, *Cone-Bearing Trees of the Pacific Coast*, p. xliii. The White Mountains are the
home of the bristlecone pines (*Pinus aristata*) and are about 20 miles northeast of Independence near the Nevada-California boundary. The trees attain an age exceeding 4,500 years
and are thought to be some of the oldest living plants.

[10]National Archives, Record Group 94, Entry 547, Book 135, pp. 263-264.

[11]"Fort Douglas Medical History," Fort Douglas Museum, Salt Lake City.

[12]Dr. T. A. Hylton is listed at Mormon Station in 1851, but it is unknown if he stayed in
the community or if he practiced medicine.

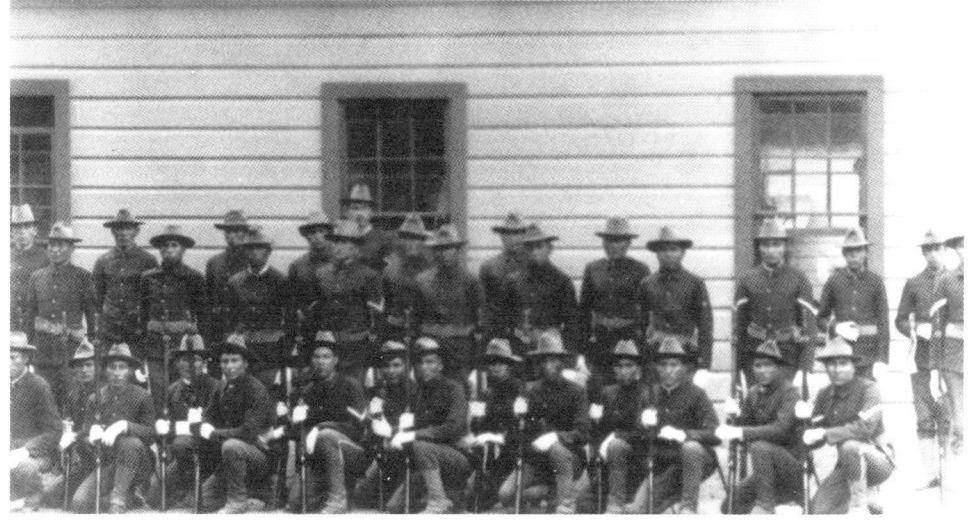

Company of Sioux Indians at Fort Douglas
Courtesy of Fort Douglas Military Museum

aged from full-time medical practice. Many were assigned by the order's leadership to work in nonmedical positions.

More importantly, the Mormon community was against the heroic ideology of regular medicine and was more closely aligned with herbal treatment, the Thomsonians. An exception was Dr. Washington R. Anderson who arrived in 1857 and became surgeon to Utah's territorial militia, the Mormon Nauvoo Legion. The scarcity of physicians in Salt Lake City came to an end in 1872, when a mining boom brought an influx of non-Mormon workers and physicians who established St. Mark's Hospital.[13]

In 1857 when Hosea Ballou Grosh died of an infected foot near Gold Canyon on the eastern side of the Great Basin —close to the future site of Virginia City, Nevada, and within twenty miles of Genoa—there were only two doctors,

[13]Bush, *Health and Medicine among the Latter-day Saints: Science, Sense, and Scripture*, pp. 93-94.

Charles D. Daggett and Benjamin L. King, in the area. The situation changed drastically with the Comstock Lode silver discoveries in June 1859. This and other mining strikes in the territory brought an influx of physicians—European, American, and Chinese—along with miners and settlers. A year later, the census of the territory listed 6,857 non-Indians, including twenty-three doctors, living in the mining districts of the western Great Basin—or one doctor per 298 persons when the national average was one per 572.[14] Indeed, in New York City there were approximately 1,500 physicians, a combination of regular, homeopathic and other practitioners, producing a ratio of one physician to each 500 inhabitants.[15] In the North before the Civil War the ratio was 1 to 595 persons, while in the South it was 1 to 526. On the wide-open and unsettled frontier there was a larger percentage of individuals calling themselves doctor which produced a ratio of 1 to 417.[16]

Several factors produced this higher concentration of doctors in the territory which would become Nevada. Some physicians came west to establish medical practice in the new towns and communities while others, forced out of practice by the uncertain economic situation back home, sought an opportunity to "strike it rich" in the mines. Due to the poor economic situation of nineteenth-century medical practice most physicians of that era frequently had another occupation; many owned pharmacies. Though trained to be physicians, in the mining camps they were simply miners or were both prospectors and part-time practitioners.

One physician attracted by the glitter of gold was Dr.

---

[14]Ibid., p. 74-75. Also see Rosen, *The Structure of American Medical Practice 1874-1941*, p. 14-15. The 23 physicians were all Euro-American. Chinese physicians were not listed in the 1860 census.

[15]Rosenberg, *Explaining Epidemics and Other Studies in the History of Medicine*, p. 127.

[16]Ackerknecht, *Malaria in the Upper Mississippi Valley 1760-1900*, p. 10.

[17]Kirkpatrick manuscript in the Bancroft Library.

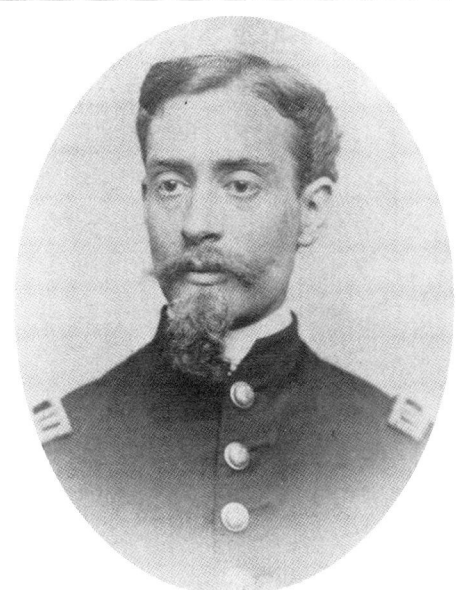

Army Doctor
Benjamin Franklin Pope
Courtesy of National Library
of Medicine

Charles A. Kirkpatrick of Grafton, Illinois, and who later served at Fort Ruby and Fort Douglas.[17] In his diary he stated:

> I was caught in the whirlpool of excitement and on the morning of the 23rd of March 1849 I turned my face to the west and took up my line of march toward the setting sun and the land of gold.... I remained on the "bar" mining and practicing medicine, as I had my sign nailed not "to the mast" but to my tent pole.
>
> When I had no patients I spent my time "rocking the cradle." There was no aristocracy then except the aristocracy of labor. Physicians fees at that time were from half an ounce [of gold] to all a man had.

A similar situation existed in the Army: some doctors enlisted for the excitement of the West while others joined because they could not make a living in their home community. Assistant Surgeon Benjamin Franklin Pope who served

[18]National Archives, RG 94, E 561.

at Camp Halleck in eastern Nevada stated that he "left private practice because there was too little of it."[18] The situation on the western frontier was about to change.

In the 1850s and '60s, a series of events changed the West and the country. Throughout the West, Native Americans reacted more boldly to the encroachment upon their lands. At that time, an estimated 7,000 to 8,500 Native Americans lived in Nevada, slightly outnumbering the new immigrants.[19] In addition the topics of polygamy and slavery were becoming more heated. The slavery issue was driving a wedge *errata*

---

[19]Train, Henrichs and Archer, *Medicinal Uses of Plants by Indian Tribes of Nevada*, p. 9.

The Great Basin Pre-War and Civil War Forts 1857-1865

PRELUDE TO FORT CRITTENDEN (THE MORMON WAR)

In 1847 the Mormon people entered the Great Salt Lake valley and established the "Mormon Kingdom," but problems related to their practice of polygamy and relationships between church and state would doom their efforts for independence. These issues were a heated, political football in Washington. After James Buchanan was elected president, a secret directive was given to General Winfield Scott ordering a march against the Mormons to prevent their founding of an independent state, thereby provoking the "Mormon War."

Captain Stewart Van Vliet in 1857 informed Brigham Young that the government planned to create the Utah Military Department and establish a military camp in the vicinity of Salt Lake City.[1] The Mormons girded for battle and refused military passage though the territory. They took the initiative and marched on Fort Bridger, burning Army provision, two wagon trains, and the fort. In disarray and with the loss of three thousand head of cattle, the Army spent a miserable winter at the burned-out fort.[2]

Reinforcements were sent to the beleaguered troops, however cooler heads prevailed and a peace commission was sent to Salt Lake City with a presidential proclamation of

[1]Moorman with Sessions, *Camp Floyd and the Mormons: The Utah War*, p. 23.
[2]Ibid., p.28.

amnesty for previous hostile actions. Brigham Young reluctantly agreed to the Army's presence in the territory. On June 26, 1858, soldiers marched through the silent and deserted streets of Salt Lake City to forever change the history of Utah and Mormondom, and erect Camp Floyd.

FORT CRITTENDEN

Camp Floyd, named for John Buchanan Floyd, Secretary of War under President James Buchanan, was built in 1857. Equidistant (forty miles) from Salt Lake City and Provo, it was "within striking distance of Fillmore City, the Territorial Capitol."[3] The Army changed the name of the camp to Fort Crittenden on February 6, 1861, when Secretary Floyd resigned after an illegal government transaction.[4] He subsequently defected to the Confederacy. It was the first fort in the Great Basin and became the fort of exploration. From its walls, the first military expeditions since Captain John C. Fremont were sent to develop new transportation routes.

Two unsuccessful expeditions were sent out, one to the Columbia River Dalles and another to the Santa Fe trail. In 1858 an expedition was launched into what would become Nevada. The health of that 1858 expedition into the Ruby Valley was overseen by Assistant Surgeon Charles Brewer.

The next major expedition occurred in 1859 when Captain James Hervey Simpson explored a new and shorter route from Camp Floyd (Salt Lake City) to Carson City and Genoa. The party of sixty-four was accompanied by Assistant Surgeon Joseph C. Baily and Private Thatcher, the hospital steward. Simpson's route became the pony express trail and later, the famous Highway 50, the "Loneliest Road" in the United States.[5] Twenty days after leaving Camp Floyd,

---

[3]Hance and Warr, *Johnston, Connor, and The Mormons*, p. 20.
[4]John Jordan Crittenden was a United States Senator from Kentucky.
[5]Simpson, *Report of Explorations across the Great Basin . . .* , p. 44.

Dr. Baily treated eight men for "a species of Intermittent fever."[6] The following day the expedition leader, Captain Simpson, reported in his diary:

> In cleaning out the spring, where we have encamped, the bones of a human being were found far-gone in decomposition. This is corroborative of the statement of my guide, last fall, that the Indians of this region bury their dead frequently in springs. It may be imagined that those who had drunk of the water did not feel very comfortable after the discovery. Fortunately for my mess the cook had used the water from the kegs which had been filled at the last camp.[7]

In appreciation for the doctors who served at Camp Floyd, Simpson named springs on the trail for Drs. Thomas H. Williams and Charles Brewer.

Other military surgeons assigned to the fort, Drs. Kirtley Ryland, Roberts Bartholow, and John Moore were also involved in exploring and taking the first recorded scientific measurements, consisting of meteorological data and a description of flora, fauna, and geology, in the Great Basin.[8]

PRELUDE TO FORT CHURCHILL
(THE LAKE PYRAMID WAR)

In late April and early May 1860, one year after the explorations from Camp Floyd, the Paiutes, one of the major tribes in the vicinity of the Comstock, met at Pyramid Lake with some of their allies, including some of the more aggressive Bannocks. The meeting was called to decide on action to protect their hunting, fishing and pine-nut gathering territories from the five thousand recently arrived miners.[9] In spite

---

[6]Ibid., p. 72.

[7]Ibid., p. 73. The expedition also recorded other situations where the Indians were not concerned about personal hygiene. They noted immense piles of feces in front of their wicke-ups (conical stick shelters). Ibid., p. 56.

[8]Ryland was temporarily at Fort Floyd when he was stationed at Fort Bridger which is outside the Great Basin.

[9]Varley, *Brigham and the Brigadier*, p. 41.

of wise council for moderation by some of the elders, a subsequent event brought war and the establishment of more forts in the Great Basin.

Two young Northern Paiute girls went out to dig for roots and didn't return. Later, Numa, a member of the tribe, went to Williams' Station and was involved in a trade dispute when he heard the girls cry out. On May 7, 1860, he returned with other members of the tribe and demanded the girls. After rescuing the kidnapped girls a fight broke out; two white men were killed and another drowned in the river. Williams' Station, located near the future site of Fort Churchill, was burned and the largest battle in the future territory of Nevada ensued.[10]

A hastily assembled and ill-advised group of 105 men from Virginia [City], Genoa, Carson City, and Silver City set out for the Paiute stronghold at Lake Pyramid to punish the encamped Indians. The group was poorly organized and had no leader, even though Major William M. Ormsby of the Carson City Rangers is often spoken of as their leader. In the expedition were two physicians, Russian-born Anton William Tjader and William E. Eichelroth.[11] On May 12, this novice group of Comstock warriors fled after the hostile Paiutes and their allies killed seventy-six, including the Major Orsmby.[12]

---

[10]Eben, Emm, and Nez, *Numa: A Northern Paiute History*, pp. 27-29. Also see Egan, *Sand in a Whirlwind: The Paiute Indian War of 1860,* and Leland, ed. *Frederick West Lander: A Biographical Sketch.*

[11]Angel, ed., *History of Nevada,* p. 153.

[12]The Regular Army clashes with Indians in Nevada, not including the Pyramid Lake War, were in the two year period of 1866-1868. According to Heitman there were 11 officially recognized skirmishes, mostly in the Fort McDermit area, but they were all minor when compared to the Pyramid Lake action. Heitman, *Historical Register and Dictionary of the United States Army,* pp. 405-31. On the other hand, the fieriest Indian battles in the Great Basin were fought in Utah. (The 1873 Modoc Indian War in the lava beds of northeastern California were outside of the Great Basin, but troops from the Great Basin participated.) The battle in Utah at Bear River and the Mountain Meadows Massacre are mentioned in a later chapter.

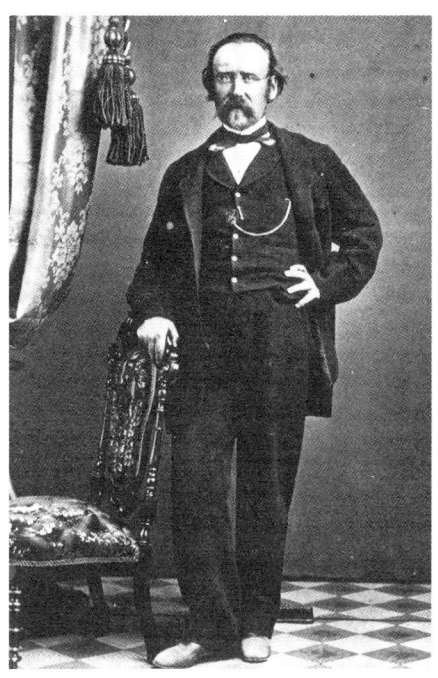

Doctor Anton William
Tjader, Nevada Militia
Courtesy of Nevada State Museum

The newly established citizens in the vicinity dug in. Temporary battle stations were hurriedly built during the panic that swept the western Great Basin. By May 15 soldiers had established a small earthen fortress named Camp Haven on the nearby Truckee River. The first patient treated by the camp surgeon at Camp Haven that day was Army Sergeant Walsh, diagnosed as suffering from intermittent fever (malaria). The camp, named after Major General J. P. Haven of the California Militia who accompanied the expedition, existed until the army built Fort Churchill later in the year.

On May 17, five days after the debacle, Dr. Anton Tjader, who had been listed as killed and scalped, stumbled to safety at Virginia City. He had enlisted as a volunteer surgeon with the Carson City Rangers, a group formed to fight at Pyramid. He was the last man to return from the battle.[13]

After the news of the Pyramid Lake massacre spread through California and across the nation, soldiers rushed across the Sierra Nevada range while frightened citizens in the vicinity of the Comstock fled to California for safety. The California troops, known as "The Carson Valley Expedition," had one surgeon, Captain Charles C. Keeney. As a result of this reinforcement, a mixed military-civilian company of over 700 men was able to rout and kill an estimated 160 Indians in the vicinity of Pyramid Lake on June 2.[14]

The company, in addition to Keeney, included physicians Edward T. Perkins and Rezin Bell. Dr. Edmund Gardner Bryant, a cousin of Poet William Cullen Bryant, was a surgeon with the company, but he found a substitute, most likely Bell or Perkins (no other physicians are known to have accompanied the troops), to represent him before he retreated to the safety of Virginia City.[15]

After the defeat, sporadic reprisals against settlements continued throughout the area. The Shoshone, Paiute and Utes threatened travelers, residents and the newly established Pony Express. This necessitated a firm and quick United States Government military strategy. On July 13, 1860, Special Order No. 67 from the Adjutant General's Office in California created Fort Churchill, the first constructed fort in the western Great Basin.[16] From that date until 1893 when the army abandoned Fort Bidwell, over

---

[13]Gary N. Tjader of Los Altos, California.

[14]The exact number of causalities the Indians suffered is not known and the estimates vary considerably. The number of 160 killed is from Angel, ed., *History of Nevada*, p. 162.

[15]Ibid., p. 159. Also see, Lewis, *Silver Kings*, p. 72-73; and Berlin, *Silver Platter*. Bryant's participation is mentioned in a letter to his father—see appendix II.

[16]National Archives RG 94, *Orders and Special Orders from the Adjutant General's Office, Department of California, 1860.*

forty camps, posts or forts were established in the western Great Basin, but many, unoccupied or occupied only a few weeks, left few records. Of these, Churchill, Nye, Ruby, McDermit, McGarry, Scott, and Halleck in Nevada; Independence and Bidwell in California; Warner and Harney in Oregon; and Three Forks in Idaho were the most important and staffed with doctors—designated surgeons or assistant surgeons by the army.[17] All but two, Nye and McGarry, are known to have had a building designated as a hospital.[18]

In the eastern Great Basin small temporary camps and larger posts were also built to cope with hostilities from Indians in the territory. Three posts—Crittenden, Rawlins, and Douglas—were located near Salt Lake City while Cameron was located to the south, near the center of Utah. These and the western Great Basin forts were established along the trails and principal lines of transportation. The concept of the frontier along a north-south line had been outdated for 20 years; the new forts were more strategically located to protect travelers.

Also the fort designed as a defensive stockade was no longer tenable. Constructed to carry out offensive missions, the Great Basin forts also had a defensive function. They protected and fed friendly Native Americans living in the vicinity of the fort.

Featuring an open central parade ground with a prominent flag pole, the typical Great Basin fort was constructed with buildings on four sides. The officers, administrative buildings, the post surgeon and usually the hospital were situated prominently at the top of the quadrangle. (In later years the hospital was isolated several hundred yards from the quadrangle.) Located on another side of the parade grounds

---

[17]Fort Three Forks is outside of the Great Basin as defined by the boundaries on the earlier map, however since it is on the brim and its soldiers patrolled south into the Basin I have included it in this work.

[18]National Archives, RG 94, E 547, B 347.

were the enlisted men and their barracks, but they were obviously lower in the hierarchy. The mess and some storage buildings were also assigned to another side of the quadrangle, but less important structures were moved to the periphery, not adjacent to the parade grounds.

All Great Basin forts might be considered temporary posts by today's standards, but when they were built they were considered permanent.[19] They were usually built of local materials that were readily available. In many desert areas unbaked adobe or mud was the only abundant material. Whitewash was added to weather proof the exterior. Furthermore with the threat of winter weather and hostilities, the buildings were usually hastily "thrown together." As a result, the structures were potential and real sources of disease, morbidity, and mortality.

This potential for disease was readily recognized by the Army. Assistant Surgeon John S. Billings considered the barracks or living quarters, the guard house, and the hospital to be the most important buildings for stressing proper hygiene. He emphasized "exposure, plan, construction, and mode of heating and ventilation" along with locality to reduce the potential for disease.[20] However, location of the post was also essential to carry out the mission of the Army.

---

[19]In nineteenth century America there were four classes of military installations. First were the permanent fortifications located for security in the harbors and along the seaboard. None of the forts on the Great Basin filled this defense need. Posts of the second class were constructed during times of crises to process and train new recruits before shipping them to the battle fields. Fort Nye, constructed during the Civil War, fits into this class. Posts of the third class were the frontier forts that were intended to be permanent. Although called "forts" or "camps" they were built to accommodate less than six companies. Most of the bases in the Great Basin fulfilled this definition. The last class were the temporary posts established in the wake of present Indian hostilities and only lasted until the crises was resolved. Many such battlements were constructed in the Great Basin, but they are not enumerated in this book. Furthermore, they were usually garrisoned by troops and doctors from nearby permanent forts. Several of the bases described on the Great Basin probably started out as a temporary base and became permanent. *Circular No. 4. A Report on Barracks and Hospitals . . .*, p. xv.

[20]Ibid., p. vi.

Location on transportation routes, an important consideration in location of the bases, resulted in the convenient location of medical facilities for civilian use. So situated, the assigned surgeon and hospital provided emergency medical services for travelers and settlers. These new hospitals featured contemporary principles of design and construction that was undergoing a metamorphosis and reflected the latest theory of disease in the nineteenth century.

Using principles of hygiene and sanitation, the military hospitals on the Great Basin featured multiple sources of ventilation. A supply of fresh, adequate air free from impurities was considered the highest priority of a good hospital. Fresh air that exceeded by 25 percent the necessary amount thought to be needed for a well person was considered a minimum for a patient on a hospital ward. For a male three thousand cubic feet of fresh air per hour was considered necessary for most diseases, but febrile diseases increased the demand.

In order to provide this amount of fresh air, it was calculated by the Army that a ward should be twenty-four feet wide and fifteen feet high with windows on each side. Furthermore, there should be one window reaching nearly to the ceiling for every two beds.[21] Besides ventilation provided by windows, doors, fireplaces, and transoms, it was considered necessary to have verandas and gardens around the hospital so that patients could have the benefit of fresh vegetables and fresh air for recuperation.[22]

In addition to adequate ventilation, the miasma theory of disease was factored into the design of the hospitals. The theory took into consideration that organic effluvia were given off from the bodies and excreta of the sick. Emissions of organic gases arose from dressings, poultices and soiled clothing causing building materials and objects within the hospital ward to absorb organic matter. In addition, organic

[21]Ibid., p. xxi.   [22]Parkes, *A Manual of Practical Hygiene,* v. II, pp. 6-8.

substances from the bedding, clothing, water-closets, and urinals added to the organic vapors. In some situations whole walls of hospitals were replaced because they had absorbed disease producing vapors and were thought to be the origin of contagious gangrene.[23]

To decrease the buildup of organic matter small wards of twenty to thirty patients were considered more healthful than larger wards. To further decrease the absorption of organic vapors the walls and floors were sealed with paint and wax.[24] These theories did not benefit from the knowledge of bacteria, but they were not far off the mark. The floors, walls and objects in modern twentieth-century hospitals can harbor disease producing staphylococcus and other bacteria.

Unfortunately, many of the early military hospitals on the Great Basin did not take advantage of these theories of ventilation and contagion. They were hurriedly constructed, sometimes using tents, dugouts, sod buildings, and even caves to provide wards for the sick before winter arrived. These crude structures were often used for several years before they were replaced. In 1858, the Army built the first military hospital in the Great Basin at Fort Crittenden, while the first described hospital in the western Great Basin was built at Fort Churchill in 1860. These structures were built to last no more than fifteen years because the buildup of organic vapors was considered a danger and a threat to health.

FORT CHURCHILL

Fort Churchill was ideally situated close to the junction of both the California and Central Overland trails from the east, and the Walker River and Carson Pass trails to the west. Forty-one miles from Carson City, it was named by Captain Joseph Stewart to honor General Sylvester Churchill (1783-1862), Inspector General of the U. S. Army and hero of the

---

[23]Ibid.   [24]Ibid.

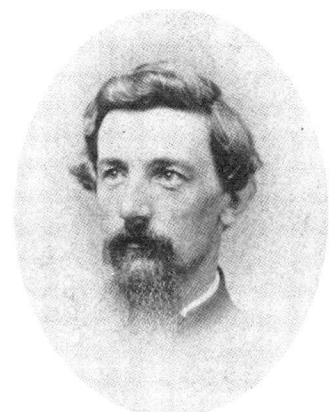

Army Doctor John Jefferson Milhau
Courtesy of National Library of Medicine

Mexican War. This base not only shielded settlers from the native peoples, but was also a force for the Union during the Civil War. On occasion, troops from the fort were called to Virginia [City], Washoe City or Carson City, all hot-beds of Southern sympathy, fostered partly by Tennessee-born Dr. Sheldon McMeans who practiced in Virginia [City].[25]

Once, McMeans organized a group of two hundred southern secessionists to support the Confederacy.[26] For punishment the southern sympathizers were taken to Fort Churchill and put to hard labor until they signed a loyalty oath.

While the construction of Fort Churchill was underway, Assistant Surgeon John Jefferson Milhau established a temporary clinic and admitted his first patients, Privates Boody and Seiger, on July 3, 1860. Boody had acute rheumatism, a common disease on the frontier, and Seiger suffered with acute diarrhea, another common aliment.[27] Because of the increasing hostilities and with winter approaching, the fort

---

[25]See Paher, ed., *Fort Churchill*, for activities at Fort Churchill during the Civil War.
[26]Smith, "The Sagebrush Soldiers," p.12.

was built quickly. In late October or early November 1860, troops and civilian construction workers, finished the hospital: an "L"-shaped sixty-three by sixty-eight feet adobe building with twenty-inch walls and twelve-foot ceilings.[28]

In order to complete the hospital before severe weather set in and to prevent further cost overruns, Lieutenant Milhau compromised with the commanding officer and down-scaled the plan for the building.[29] The original fort was to be modestly built of readily procured materials, but expensive materials were being used, including lumber from California and supplies from Virginia [City]. A board of investigation found some of the buildings to be too elaborate and cutbacks were ordered. Milhau argued for the original hospital and lost. The compromised hospital's exact size of the wards and number of beds is not known, but it contained at least four rooms, a cellar and three fireplaces.[30] It is unlikely that the ward contained more than a recommended twenty to thirty beds. During its existence Fort Churchill, the largest of the Nevada military installations, garrisoned up to six hundred men and sent many east to serve in the Civil War.

Initially, commissioned officers who were regular army doctors, designated assistant surgeons or surgeons with the rank of lieutenant or captain, commanded the hospital; but later civilian (contract) doctors, designated acting assistant surgeons, attended the soldiers. In all, fifteen doctors served at Fort Churchill.[31] In contrast to smaller military posts in the Great Basin, the hospital at Fort Churchill during its first year of existence was well staffed with stewards, and sometimes two doctors.

---

[27]National Archives, RG 94, *Hospital Records of Fort Churchill.*

[28]National Archives, RG 92, E 225.   [29]Ibid.

[30]The ruins show foundations dividing the building into four distinct rooms. Obviously, these rooms could have been further partitioned.

[31]National Archives, M 617, *Returns from U. S. Military Posts 1800-1916,*. The army started using civilian doctors toward the end of the Civil War and Abel F. Mechem, at Fort Churchill in 1864, was the first contract doctor in Nevada.

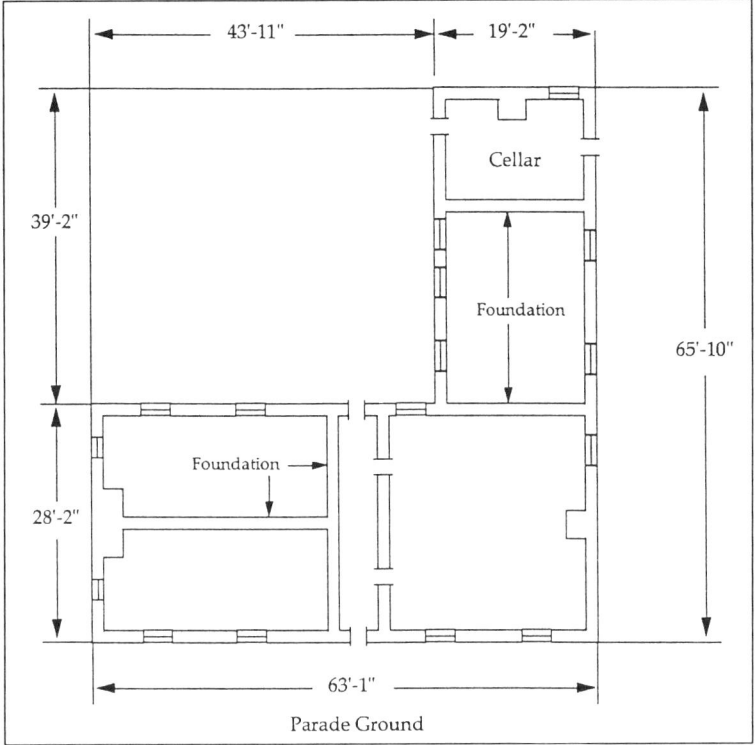

Plan of Fort Churchill's Hospital, 1860
Drawing by author and Anton Phillip Sohn

CLOSURE OF FORT CRITTENDEN

On July 21, 1861, after the defeat at Bull Run, the Army moved all regular units east.[32] Six days later Fort Crittenden closed. During its brief period of existence it served as a stop on the Pony Express and Central Overland Stage Route, a line of defense against the Mormons, and a staging point for exploring the Great Basin.[33] In its four years of existence

---

[32]Smith, "The Sagebrush Soldiers," pg. 11.

[33]Chapman, *The Pony Express*, pp. 90, 290. The Pony Express existed less than two years, from April 1860 until Oct. 1861.

eighty-four soldiers were buried in the base cemetery prompting one soldier to poetically describe the medical condition at the fort:

> The state of health in camp is very low, and every day we hear the solemn notes of the dead march, and the roll of musketry over the grave of some poor fellow who has ended his earthly career in this distant region, far from the soothing hands of kind relatives. It is sad to see the sick lying upon their beds, with no one to soothe their pillows but rough soldiers, whose awkward attempts to be gentle almost excite a smile in the midst of sorrow. Thank Heaven, I have, as yet, borne up well, and I hope that Providence will carry me safely though, that my dying hours may be amid more genial scenes and my last rites performed by gentler hands.[34]

By now the Civil War was going badly for the Union. Not only did President Lincoln need to secure the West and its vast resources, but its man power was needed for the Union Army. Furthermore, many westerners were anxious and willing to fight for their country. From the gold fields of California and the mining districts of Nevada Territory volunteers enlisted for the Union cause. Fort Churchill, a strategically located relay station on the route east, quickly filled to capacity with new recruits. This forced the Army to build a number of new posts in 1862 as described below.

CAMP NYE

The existence of Camp Nye could be described as a little known chapter in Nevada history. In fact, its location was only recently identified by William O'Connell of Reno. The camp honored James W. Nye, appointed Territorial Governor of Nevada and commander-in-chief of the Nevada Militia by President Abraham Lincoln. Located at the mouth of Kings Canyon near Carson City, Camp Nye had, on occasion, as many as 230 men. The records name only Acting

---

[34]Langley, ed., *To Utah With the Dragoons . . .*, p. 129.

Assistant Surgeons George Munckton and William Octavus Eversfield during its existence, June 1862 to August 1865. (There are no records for May through August 1865.)[35] No known description of the post hospital remains, but as was true for most urgently needed forts, the order to build the post included a temporary tent hospital.

FORT INDEPENDENCE

Fort Independence was established on Independence Day, July 4, 1862, to quell Owens Valley Paiute disturbances and to protect settlers on the fertile farm land of the Owens Valley.[36] Located at the southwestern corner of the Great Basin at the foot of Mount Whitney, the highest peak in the continental United States, the fort's hospital and doctors provided important health services to area residents. The first hospital at Independence might have been in a cave since the soldiers spent the first winter in caves near the future site of the fort.[37] In 1862 when the Army arrived, there were 1,700-2,000 Owens Valley Paiutes, but by the time they left in 1877 there were approximately 900 and, in 1887 the population had decreased to 776.[38]

The military camp at Independence was prematurely abandoned for a short time in 1864 after the Army in a poorly thought out order moved one thousand Paiutes from Owens Valley to Fort Tejon, California. With renewed hostilities, Fort Independence reopened early in 1865. In September of that year, Assistant Surgeon Charles C. Keeney was sent to establish a new hospital.

In addition to its previous mission, the post became a staging base for the Wheeler mapping expedition which official-

---

[35]National Archives, M 617.

[36]*Handbook of North American Indians*, v. 11, Great Basin, p. 430.

[37]Hart, *Old Forts of the Far West*, p. 42.

[38]Cragen, *The Boys in the Sky-Blue Pants*, p. 187. According to William Michaels at the Eastern California Museum the population is now between 1,200 and 1,300.

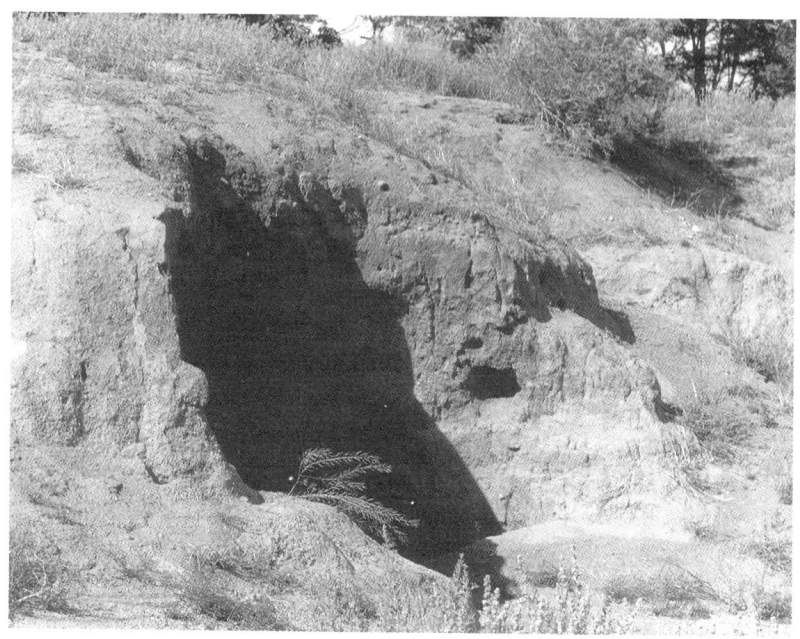

Caves at Fort Independence
Photograph by the author

ly began at Fort Halleck in 1872. Lieutenant George M. Wheeler headed the military expedition with orders to develop topographical maps with mineral deposits and geological formations. Two doctors, Adam H. Cochrane and A. H. Hoffman, were in the party.[39] Hoffman, a naturalist, collected two thousand beetles and discovered several new butterfly species while at Fort Independence.[40]

Nonetheless, medical practice at the fort was more important to the inhabitants of Owens Valley than the gathering of scientific information and natural history. In 1875, an epidemic of scarlet fever killed three children in one family and several more in the community. Dr. J. D. Blair, a new civilian arrival in the valley, treated the illness with "success." The

[39]Ibid., p. 93. In *The Inyo Independent*, July 22, 1871, Hoffman stated "the primary object of [the survey] is a full and complete report of the geology, entomology, fauna and flora of these regions."   [40]Cragen, *The Boys in the Sky-Blue Pants*, p. 95.

Paiute inhabitants also suffered from epidemics and were treated by military doctors after they killed their medicine men whom the Indians accused of witchcraft.[41]

In addition to scarlet fever, epidemics of measles and smallpox swept the Owens Valley in 1876 and '77. By September 3, 1876, Indians in Bishop, Banyon, and Round Valley were infected with measles. Mike Bishop and other Indian medicine men were put to death by their people for failure to invoke a cure, but the epidemic continued through the winter. As it disappeared from the upper valley the disease "hit" the community of Big Pine. Four or five more medicine men were killed. In November it became obvious that the Indian doctors couldn't stop the "contagion." Dr. Blair ordered them to cease sweat lodges and cold plunges.[42]

The tribe held the shamans accountable and during the epidemic killed more than eighty of their medicine men and their sons for practicing witchcraft.[43] Thus, many of their healing traditions were lost and little is known of their medical practices. Early in the epidemic Dr. Washington Matthews from nearby Fort Independence offered help, but the Owens Valley Paiute were suspicious of non-native medicine. The following year a smallpox epidemic hit the Owens Valley and they were now desperate for help.

Indian guide Joe Bowers requested help for his Deep Springs tribe. The fort commander authorized vaccination for "25¢ a head." Lieutenant Wotherspoon took vaccination supplies to the community and Dr. Matthews vaccinated all Indians who came in for help. A local citizen, A. N. Bell, brought in thirty Indians and forty more were vaccinated by the medical team on a trip up the valley. By March 17 Matthews had vaccinated two hundred.[44]

---

[41]Ibid., p. 168.
[42]*The Inyo Independent*, Aug. 19, 1876; Sept. 3 and 9, Nov. 11, and Dec. 9, 1876.
[43]Cragen, *The Boys in the Sky-Blue Pants*, p. 184.
[44]*The Inyo Independent*, March 3, 10, and 17, 1877.

FORT RUBY

When Fort Independence was founded in 1862 the Civil War was at its height. Volunteers were joining the colors in California and Nevada hoping to be sent to the Army of the Potomac. Colonel Patrick Edward Connor was selected to command the volunteers from the Mother Lode. Colonel Conner established Fort Ruby in September 1862. Conner and his troops arrived in the Ruby Valley during an early winter snow storm. Fort Ruby was located at the foot of the spectacular Ruby Mountains which had been named by early settlers who found ruby red agates in a canyon above the valley floor. Construction time was short and timber was scarce so the buildings were dug four feet into the ground. The fort provided a way-station for volunteers on the way to the Civil War, but it was also situated to protect travelers on the Overland stage route. Soon after construction there were problems with discipline and morale. Not only was the post crudely built and located on a remote desert, but its troops were not permitted to go east and participate in the war for which they had volunteered. Assistant Surgeon Isaac W. Brown who served at the post exemplified the problems that plagued the post.

Army personnel records indicate that in 1864 Dr. Brown and two other lieutenants were arrested and forced to resign.[45] Although a fire destroyed the hospital and its records on November 14, 1868, the details of Brown's dishonor are spelled out in the records of the Adjutant General's Office.[46] He violated the 25th Article of War by accepting a

---

[45]National Archives, M 617. Brown was one of several California doctors who served in Nevada. Some were assistant surgeons in the California Volunteers and were not commissioned in the U. S. Army. At the end of the Civil War they were mustered out of the army. Others were civilians who signed contracts and served at the Nevada bases. In addition to Brown the California physicians at Great Basin forts included Cassell, Furley, Gwyther, Handy, Hayes, Kirkpatrick, Reid, Ramatke and Woods. For a complete listing of California physicians in the Civil War see Hunt, *The Army of the Pacific, 1860-1866*, pp. 279-80.

[46]National Archives, RG 94, E 544 and RG 94, *Records of the Adjutant's General's Office*.

challenge and fighting a duel with Second Lieutenant Edward Ingham. Afterwards, the commanding officer, Lieutenant Colonel J. B. Moore, discovered that the duel "was a Sham, that the Pistols were loaded with Powder and Cotton, and that his [Brown's] object was to do something that he might get his discharge from the service."[47] In spite of the fact that Moore recommended Brown be punished, he was allowed to resign. Like so many of the other Great Basin army physicians he vanished into history along with the buildings of the fort. Today only a log cabin, probably the sutler's store, and a small stone structure near the spring remain at the site of Fort Ruby which is known as Andy's Fort Ruby Ranch.

FORT DOUGLAS

After leaving troops for security and to construct Fort Ruby, Conner proceeded to Salt Lake City by stage to assess the situation. He was offered the abandoned Fort Crittenden for the outrageous sum of $15,000. Realizing that it would be difficult to rebuild a fort at the Fort Crittenden site for want of accessible timber, Connor elected to build a new fort against the demands of the Mormon leadership on a plateau three miles above Salt Lake City. He returned with his men and established Fort Douglas.

The forts on the western slope of the Wasatch Mountains of Utah were some of the largest in the West. Fort Critten-den on occasion had three thousand men and was the largest military garrison.[48] Even Fort Douglas with fifteen hundred men was larger than any other Great Basin fort.[49] Colonel Conner's stated purpose in Salt Lake City was to secure the mail lines and immigration trails from the Indians, but in addition, he was instructed to guarantee the loyalty of the Mormon settlement.

---

[47]Ibid.   [48]Hart, *Old Forts of the Far West*, pp. 173-74.
[49]Caum, "Fort Douglas, Utah," p. 6.

The fear of a Mormon insurrection against the United States government was bolstered by the past hostile actions of the Mormon armed guards, including the burning of three wagon trains and Fort Bridger. To prevent further hostile Mormon activity Connor's unit included one thousand infantry, five hundred cavalry, and two howitzers, along with three ambulances, a regimental band, dependents, and Surgeon Robert Reid.

Opposed by Brigham Young and out-numbered by Mormon troops, tension was high when Conner and his men advanced on Salt Lake City. The sick were asked to shoulder rifles and be prepared to fight.

> Five men were sick in the hospital and thirty-six sick in quarters. At sick call, Surgeon Reid, who had been arranging his abominable knives, saws and probes, said that this was a day when every man able to carry a musket should do so, and one that would determine who were loafers and who were soldiers. Twenty-eight out of the forty-one, many of whom were really unfit for service, shouldered their pieces, and the remainder did not, only because they could not.[50]

An armed confrontation was avoided and the men established Fort Douglas in October 1862 after marching past the Governor's residence to demonstrate their resolve. The fort, now the site of the University of Utah, became the premiere base in the Great Basin and lasted until 1991, a tenure of almost one hundred and thirty years. Several buildings, including the original morgue, remain near the parade grounds. In contrast to the barren landscape of the Great Basin, Fort Douglas was situated on the rim of the stunning Wasatch range of the Rocky Mountains. Assistant Surgeon William Cline Borden described the scene in 1885:

> From Ogden to Salt Lake City the railroad passed through a continuous succession of peach orchards in full blossom, and the air was redolent with their perfume. I remained at Fort Douglas 3

---

[50]Rogers, *Soldiers of the Overland:*, p. 48.

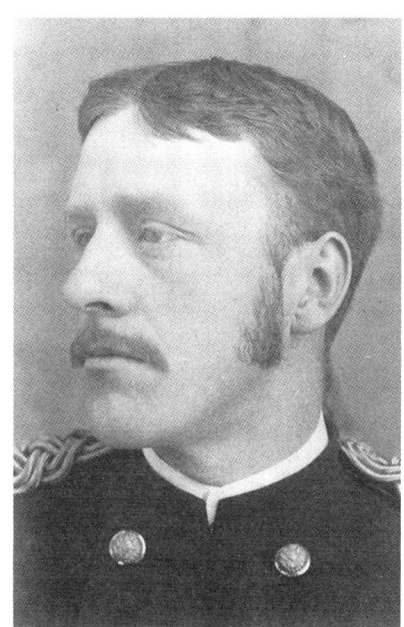

Army Doctor
William Cline Borden
Courtesy of National Library
of Medicine

years, and I look back upon this as the pleasantest station I have had since entering the army.

The Post is pleasant, the climate the finest I have ever lived in, and the scenery magnificent. From the Post situated on the western slope of the Wasatch Mountains, the valley of the Great Salt Lake with its farms and city is spread like a panorama below …[51]

Named for the deceased "Little Giant," Senator Stephen A. Douglas, one of Lincoln's opponents for President, the fort in its first thirty-eight years of existence had a succession of forty-eight physicians, including such notables as Charles Smart and William Hemple Arthur who had successful army careers and retired as generals.[52]

Hospitalization was initially provided at Fort Douglas by a

[51]Borden, "William Cline Borden 1858-1934," p. 2.

[52]It is known that Lincoln respected Douglas and he probably gave the order to name the fort after the deceased Senator.

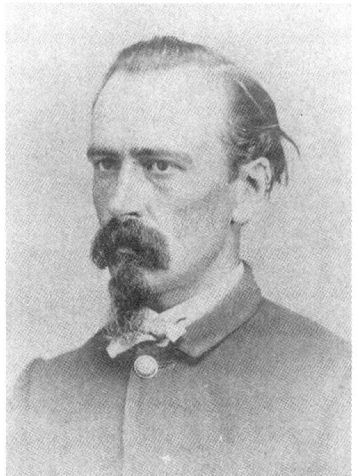
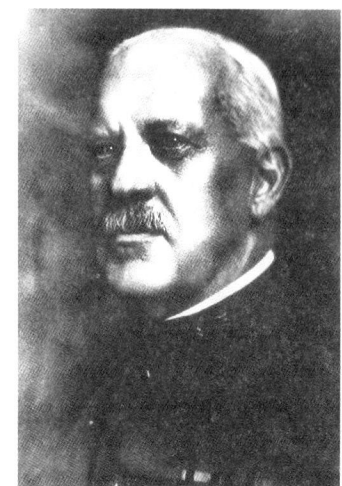

Army Doctors Charles Smart (left) and William Hemple Arthur (right)
Both photos courtesy of National Library of Medicine

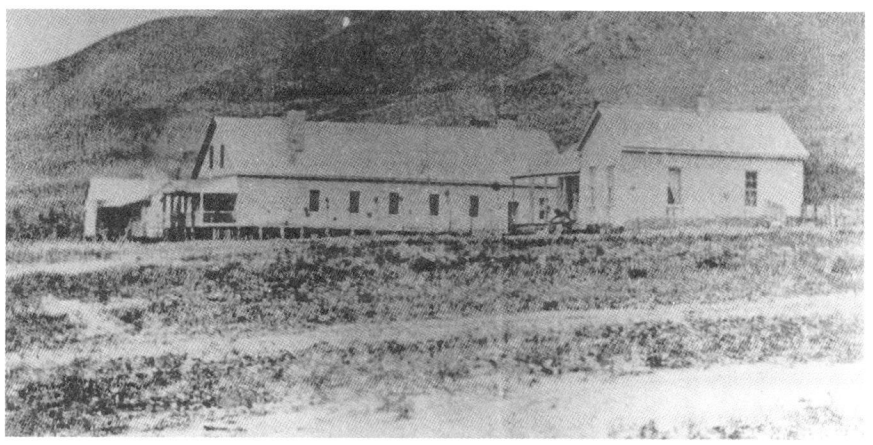

Fort Douglas Hospital with Surgeon's Quarters on the right, 1864
Courtesy of Fort Douglas Military Museum

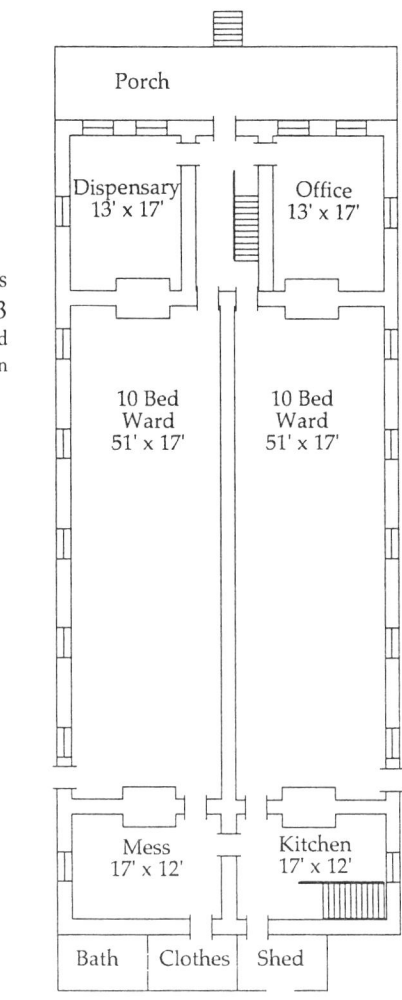

Plan of Fort Douglas
Hospital, 1863
Drawing by author and
Anton Phillip Sohn

small log cabin and three hospital tents.[53] The first permanent hospital built in October 1863, was constructed of
roughly-hewn white pine with a sandstone foundation and
covered with a shingled roof. The building was eighty-eight
by thirty-six and was twenty-seven feet high at the peak. The
interior was lathed and plastered. There were two ten-bed
wards 51 feet 3 inches by 16 feet 9 inches with two ventilat-

---

[53]Information provided by Charles G. Hibbard, Historian at the Fort Douglas Military
Museum.

ing shafts providing 858 cubic feet of air per bed. During the early years, the hospitals primary function was to care for those wounded in battle. Records indicate that there was little sickness at the fort.

> The sick and wounded receive every attention and all the luxuries the country affords. But little sickness has prevailed at the post ... [Only] wounds and injuries received on the march to and at the battle of Bear River, [resulted in hospitalization. There were] seventy sick in quarters and twenty-two in [the] hospital; one officer and six men have died of their wounds, all being shot in a vital part; four men have had their toes amputated, and two have lost a finger each. The inmates of the hospital are now doing well, and with one exception will all probably recover.[54]

From the Bear River battle which occurred in January 1863, Surgeon Robert K. Reid transported the wounded in eighteen sleighs through two feet of snow. Private Lee, transported with a leg wound, wondered if he would freeze or bleed to death. Surgeons Jonathan M. Williamson and Walcott Steele met the caravan of ambulances near Ogden to help care for the wounded. Later, Connor cited Reid for his skill and bravery. The battle was one of the most successful in the West and was more fierce and bloody than Sand Creek or Wounded Knee.[55]

Fort Douglas was established in an area that was unfamiliar to the Surgeon General prompting a letter dated October 29, 1874, asking questions about the climate's effect on a soldier's health. "What is the average pulse and respiration rate at the Post? What are the diurnal variations in temperature? What is the influence, if any, of adobe habitations on the health of the inmates?" This was of particular significance because many of the forts in the West and Southwest would be built of adobe. To answer the question Surgeon Edward

---

[54]Rogers, *Soldiers of the Overland*, p. 60.

[55]Varley, *Brigham and the Brigadier*, pp. 110-12.

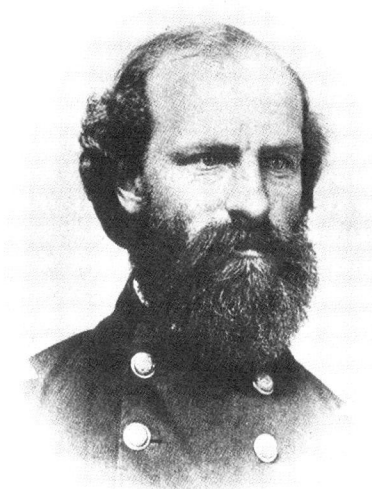

Army Doctor
Edward Perry Vollum
Courtesy of National Library
of Medicine

Perry Vollum tested twenty-five soldiers and replied that the slightly increased pulse and respiration rates found at Fort Douglas were due to the effects of tobacco. He further stated that in his experience the adobe bricks had no ill effects on the inhabitants.[56]

---

[56] *Circular No. 8*, p. 344.

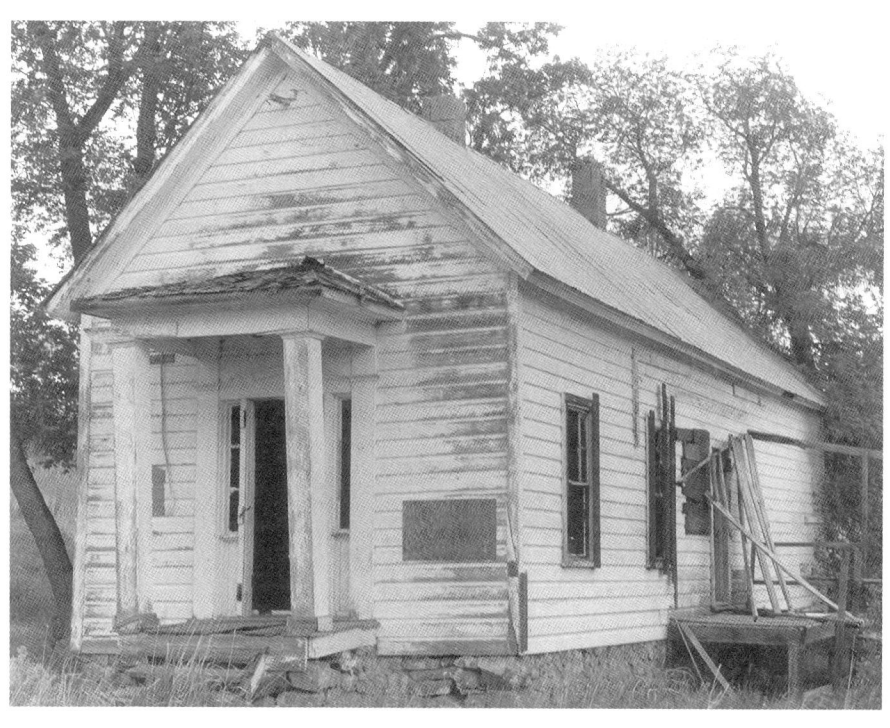

Fort Bidwell School, the only building still standing on the original site
Photograph by the author

Founding of the Great Basin Post-Civil War Forts 1865-1870

Peace was signed and the Civil War was over, now the nation could again turn its attention to its western settlements and the development of the West. Land and opportunity in the Northwest (Oregon and Washington) and California was alluring, but Indian hostilities in the Great Basin, even though on a diminished scale, were still occurring. To meet the threat, ten forts were established in the Intermountain West during the seven year period after the War.

Fort Nye, no longer necessary for training recruits to fight in the Civil War, was dismantled and the land became a private ranch. Peaceful pasture and livestock replaced the clatter and hurried motion of training troops. In other parts of Great Basin peace was still a dream. Fort Bidwell was the first postwar military base constructed in the Great Basin to moderate the hostilities between the Native Indians and the growing wave of western population.

FORT BIDWELL

John Bidwell, joined by concerned citizens of Surprise Valley, Red Bluff, Shasta, and Honey Lake, used his infulence to have the fort placed where it protected his transportation of goods from California to the Idaho mines. Military leaders agreed and placed Fort Bidwell to protect the new settlers and travelers on the Lassen-Applegate trail to Oregon and northern California.[1] Even though the heyday of western migration

on overland trails was over, it would be four years before the
railroad connecting the East with the West would be finished.
Fort Bidwell was established July 17, 1865, in Surprise Valley,
in the far northeast corner of California, an area to this day
untouched and known for its solitary and stunning beauty.
The fort was named to honor John Bidwell, a prominent early
Californian, a Mexican War veteran, a member of Congress,
and the founder of the city of Chico.[2]

To construct Fort Bidwell the Army troops took advantage of the abundant trees in the nearby mountains and constructed its first hospital from hand-hewn logs which
supported a shingled roof. Bidwell's hospital consisted of
three wings: a 27 feet by 23 feet room with a dispensary and
steward's room on the north, a 10 by 23 room for a kitchen
and mess on the south, and a 22 by 29 twelve-bed ward with
1,200 cubic feet of air per bed situated between the two.[3] In
addition the hospital had two four-acre gardens located
south of the parade ground.[4] (Only the old, decaying
school/chapel on one side of the old parade grounds is still
standing at the site of the fort.) While Fort Bidwell was
under construction, Forts McDermit and McGarry were
built in the fall and winter of 1865 to protect remote sections
of wagon and stagecoach trails.

FORT MCDERMIT

Fort McDermit guarded from 1865 to 1889 the Win-
nemucca-Boise stage route.[5] The post was located near the
Oregon border on the northeast corner of the Black Rock

---

[1]Davis, *Sagebrush Corner,* p. 101.

[2]John Bidwell was a member and secretary of the Bartleson Party as a young man in 1841,
the first group of American emigrants to travel overland to California. He attained land and
wealth in California, and in 1892 ran for President as the Prohibition Party candidate.

[3]Whiting, *Forts of the State of California,* p. 13, and Tyler, *Revised Outlines and Descriptions of Posts and Stations of Troops in the Military Division of the Pacific,* p. 19.

[4]*Circular No. 4.,* p. 446.

[5]McDermit is sometimes spelled McDermitt.

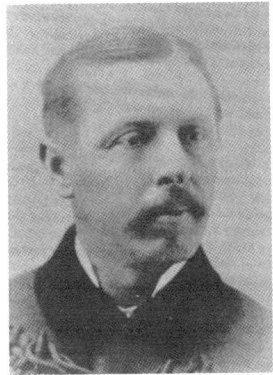

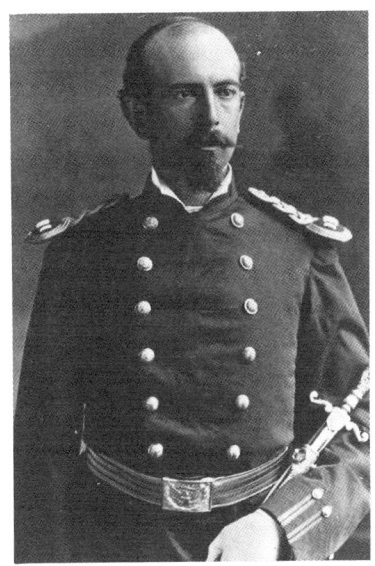

Army Doctors
George Martin Kober (above) and
William Henry Corbusier (right)
Above, courtesy of Patricia A. Barry; right,
courtesy National Library of Medicine

Desert. Fort McDermit was named to honor Lieutenant Colonel Charles McDermit killed earlier that year in the Jackson Mountains on the southeast corner of the Black Rock Desert, during action against the Northern Paiute.

In addition to the soldiers, three hundred Paiutes and Chief Winnemucca who were loyal to the government also lived at the fort. It existed for nearly twenty-four years, the longest of any Nevada fort. When it was abandoned the Department of Interior gave the buildings and land to be used as an Indian school and reservation. Only one of the original buildings, an officer's quarters, remains to this day and is used as a senior citizens center where everyone is welcomed at the weekly senior citizens' lunch. Its white-washed adobe facade is testimony to a more turbulent era.

Acting Assistant Surgeons George Martin Kober and William Henry Corbusier served at the post and kept substantial records. They later wrote of their remembrances at the desolate and lonely Nevada outpost, recalling in their journals Chief Winnemucca and his daughter, Sarah, who was a matron at the McDermit hospital.[6] They, also, described life at the fort and wrote of details about their medical practice.

Corbusier's wife, Fanny, a school teacher, kept a journal of her life on the Nevada desert. Her first description of the Nevada frontier is about their trip on July 24, 1869, to McDermit from Winnemucca, "a small collection of houses in the desert." When the Corbusiers stopped for lunch, on the way to the fort, flies were a problem. After traveling in an ambulance they spent the night at the stage "home-station." Fanny tried sleeping in the ambulance, but finally went into the house because of the howling wind and the frightening noise of the coyotes which she naively thought was a hostile tribe of Indians.

The Corbusier party arrived at McDermit at noon on Saturday, July 25. Her husband relieved Acting Assistant Surgeon George Gwyther who lost no time in returning to civilization; he left the next day. Her impressions of the post were terse. "In the middle of the parade ground was a very crooked flag staff made of three small willow trees, spliced and bound together with iron hoops.…[and] nothing green to relieve the eyes.[7]

She also noted after arrival, that the hospital was a forty feet by twenty-eight feet adobe structure with a four-bed ward. In describing her husband's duties, she related that he

[6]National Archives, RG 94, E 547. Also, Summerhayes, *Vanished Arizona*, pp. 237 and 249. Summerhayes also wrote that "Camp MacDermit was a colorless, forbidding sort of a place" and she characterized Halleck as "a lovely place." Also Hein, *Memories of Long Ago*, p. 99.

[7]Corbusier, *Verde to San Carlos:* p. 90. Corbusier's wife, Fanny Dunbar Corbusier, also wrote of her experiences in an unpublished manuscript, "Recollection of Her Life in the Army." A copy was loaned to me by Martina Ellis, Amite, Louisiana, a relative of Corbusier. The quotes from *Verde to San Carlos* are also in the unpublished manuscript.

had little to do.[8] In fact, during the long winter months there was little activity at the post and the soldiers rarely performed military functions and then, always under protest. Mrs. Corbusier related, "The men had Indians to wait on them and do all except their strictly military duties."[9]

In 1870, Drs. Corbusier and Gwyther reported to John Shaw Billings that there was no wash room or kitchen and the air space in the Fort McDermit's hospital measured 918 cubic feet per man.[10] Shortly thereafter Kober supervised construction of a new hospital.

Fort McGarry

Unlike Fort McDermit, little has been recorded by the physicians about the daily activities at Fort McGarry. Built in November 1866, at a location near Summit Lake in northwestern Nevada, the fort guarded for two years the High Rock Canyon area of the Lassen-Applegate Cutoff. Lack of settlements in the remote area and the harsh weather conditions at the high elevation made occupancy of the fort unnecessary and difficult during the winter, when the soldiers moved south to the lower Black Rock Desert and continued their surveillance from Soldier Meadows. Two buildings remain at its former site on the Soldier Meadows Ranch, but only fragmented stone walls are seen at the Summit Lake site.

---

[8]Corbusier, *Verde to San Carlos:*, p. 96.

[9]Ibid., pp. 96-7.

[10]*Circular No. 4,* p. 453. Billings was an important late nineteenth-century doctor, a chief public health authority for the Army and builder of the Surgeon General Office's library. Billings reviewed all of the Army hospitals by report and made recommendations for corrective action in *Circular No. 4.* He emphasized proper hospital construction with particular emphasis on heating and ventilation. When the Circular was published in 1870 there were few publications on the subject in the United States. As a result his name became well known to the public and medical officials. In 1875 he compiled *Circular No. 8, Report on the Hygiene of the United States Army,* which dealt extensively with the health of soldiers. Chapman, *Order Out of Chaos: John Shaw Billings and America's Coming of Age,* pp. 83-85.

Fort McGarry, named for Civil War hero, Brevet Brigadier General Edward McGarry, was the largest Nevada military reserve with land comprising seventy-five square miles. An unusual feature at the fort was the use of underground passages connecting the barn, mess, and barracks at the Summit Lake installation which provided protection from surprise Indian raids.[11]

All five surgeons assigned to Fort McGarry were civilian doctors. The first, Siegesmund Kisffy had a diploma from the University of Pesth (Hungary), a certificate from the Eastern Medical Board of Examination of New Orleans and another from the Harvard Association of New Orleans. Because he was "totally deficient in medical qualifications the army annulled his contract August 18, 1866."[12] In spite of his shortcomings it is likely that Kisffy established the first hospital at McGarry in a tent, but no description of his efforts remains.

FORT THREE FORKS OF THE OWYHEE

Fort Three Forks on the Owyhee River (originally named Camp Winthrop) was built in 1866 north of the Nevada border in Idaho. From its strategic position it protected the fertile land and settlements in the Jordan Valley and along the Owyhee River. The post located seventy-five miles northeast of Fort McDermit was usually garrisoned by a company of infantry.

Acting Assistant Surgeon Edward Colmache was the only medical officer on duty at the fort during its brief existence. He oversaw a healthy command. Only three cases of serious illness and one death occurred during the first two years of operation. Doctor Colmache described the hospital, which took six weeks to build, as a sixty-five by twenty foot building

---

[11]Mack, *History of Nevada*, p.324.
[12]National Archives, RG 94, E 561.

on the east side of the camp. The twenty-seven by eighteen foot ward had eight beds, two windows and an adjoining kitchen with mess. The Army did not allow space for a steward, dead-house, bathroom or lavatory.

FORT WINFIELD SCOTT

Post Winfield Scott also had its troubles and defective buildings that seemed to characterize Great Basin forts. Established in 1866 at the south foot of the Santa Rosa Mountains in northern Nevada, Fort Scott honored General Winfield Scott, commander of the U.S. Army during the Mexican War. The base, thirty-five miles across the mountains from Fort McDermit and located near the tiny town of Paradise Valley, was in reality not a paradise for the encamped company of soldiers. Like many other Great Basin posts it was isolated and provided only the bare necessities for existence.

Lieutenant Hein, before he served at Forts Halleck and McDermit, commanded his first troop at Fort Scott in 1870. Shortly after arriving he "was left in command . . . with a detachment of twenty-two men, many of whom were foreigners and altogether a tough lot of individuals."[13] Fort Scott's predicament was similar to many western army bases. New immigrants to America enlisted in the Army to get free travel to the West Coast, and then deserted. At the isolated Great Basin forts desertion was a common occurrence.

Hein stayed at "this dreary station till the following spring, without companions, books or papers, and only an occasional mail which was about ten days old when it reached [him], but it was most welcome, as it constituted [his] only connection with civilization." Continuing, "I was entirely snowed in during the winter, and my only neighbors were small bands

---

[13]The preponderance of foreigners in the army was characteristic of the U. S. Army before the Civil War. In fact in 1850 a majority of the enlisted men were foreign-born. One reason was the increasing numbers of poor European emigrants in the mid-nineteenth century.

of Piute Indians, and a few scattered white ranchers, who lived in the valley some miles distant."[14] Hein relates the problem with alcohol, the base surgeon, and a conflict with the local sutler:

> The enlisted men of my command were nearly all addicted to drinking to excess, and so frequently indulged, that I found it extremely difficult to enforce any proper sort of discipline at the post . . . I forbade the men from visiting his place [off base store] any longer . . . the old post surgeon suggested, that if he were permitted to issue liquor to the men occasionally, as a "ration," he might be able to diminish and control their midnight orgies.[15]

Hein took him up on his offer, but the sutler who owned the store complained, resulting in an investigation:

> . . . It was discovered by the inspector . . . that the old German doctor [Frederick Denicke[16]] had not been quite disinterested, in his scheme for the moral and physical improvement of the men, and that he had profited pecuniarily therefrom, and this disclosure resulted in his elimination from the service, shortly afterwards.[17]

Dr. Denicke was the last of six physicians who served at the fort. His departure from the service in 1871 coincided with closure of Fort Scott.

FORT WARNER

Fort Warner was established in Southeastern Oregon. The post, built on the eastern side of Hart Mountain in 1867, was named for Captain William Horace Warner who was killed in 1849 during an Indian ambush thirty miles south of where Fort Warner would be located.[18] The troops stationed at Fort

---

[14]Hein, *Memories of Long Ago*, p. 62.   [15]Ibid., p. 63.

[16]Hein does not name the German doctor in his *Memories of Long Ago*, but according to National Archives, RG 94, E 561, Denicke was the doctor on duty at the base when the event occurred.

[17]Hein, *Memories of Long Ago*, p. 64.

[18]The body of Captain Warner was never found despite searches by the military and 20th-century historians. Hart Mountain is the winter home of the largest herd of pronghorn antelope in the Great Basin.

Warner would later participate in the fierce fight with Captain Jack and his Modoc band in the nearby lava beds which are outside the Great Basin.

In 1868 the post was moved to nearby Honey Creek. The hospital at Fort Warner was constructed of logs. Assistant Surgeon Richard Powell mordantly and honestly stated that ventilation of the ward was supplemented by the "cracks in the rudely constructed building."[19] The plan of the hospital conformed to the guidelines established by the Army in *Circular No. 4*, an L-shaped structure with the ward on one side and the steward's room, surgery, mess and kitchen on the other. A wing, forty-four by twenty-four feet, housed the twelve-bed ward that allowed 986 cubic feet of air per bed.[20]

Because of the short growing season it was difficult to grow vegetables at Fort Warner. Therefore, a garden was planted in a more favorable location sixteen miles from the hospital. However, the lack of fresh vegetables in the diet resulted in eleven cases of scurvy in 1868. The mean strength at that time was 232 men. Powell further noted that the health of the command was good and most aliments yielded to simple medicines or more preferably, a warm hospital and proper diet.[21]

FORT HALLECK

While Fort Warner was built on the northwestern edge of the Great Basin, Fort Halleck, named for Henry W. Halleck who was Commander of the Military Division of the Pacific—and more importantly, General in Chief during the Civil War—was built in 1867 near Elko in middle of the Great Basin. The Army located the base on the California Trail, near the new Central Pacific Railroad. Midway between Salt

---

[19] *Circular No. 4.*, pp. 435-36.
[20] Ibid., p. 435.   [21] Ibid.

Lake City and the small town of Winnemucca, Fort Halleck guarded the mining districts and ranches around Elko. Later, using an efficient rail and telegraph system, the army could move troops quickly to deal with emergencies in the central Great Basin, thereby making Halleck obsolete.

Military emergencies were rare in Fort Halleck's jurisdiction. Life was boring enough at this post that Lieutenant Otto Hein, four years out of West Point, often would go to Halleck Station and "there board a west bound train in which I would travel until I met the east bound train, and then return by the latter to the station, and by ambulance to the Post."[22]

A tent hospital served the wounded and sick soldiers during the first winter and part of the second. Frances Boyd, the wife of an officer, recalled how she heard the cries of the wounded through the walls of her tent. On December 20, 1868, Assistant Surgeon Benjamin Franklin Pope and his predecessor, Acting Assistant Surgeon Frank S. Stirling, completed the post hospital, a forty by thirty foot adobe building with an attached thirty by twenty-four foot frame building. The structure housed an eighteen by twelve foot surgery room, an eighteen by eighteen mess, a sixteen by twelve kitchen and an eighteen by twenty-two foot main ward with ten beds. The inside of the ward was tongue and grove boards while the outside was boards and battens.[23] The hospital, less than ideally located, required water to be carried a distance of twenty yards from a reservoir to the hospital.

FORT HARNEY

Camp Steele was originally established August 16, 1867, on Rattlesnake Creek in Southeast Oregon near the future town of Burns and a short ride from Fort Warner. The name

---

[22]Hein, *Memories of Long Ago:*, p. 101.   [23]National Archives, RG 94, E 547.

was changed to Fort Harney one month later.[24] The fort named for Mexican War hero, General William Selby Harney, was the military headquarters for action against the hostile Bannock Indians in the area. The mean strength in 1868 one year after construction of the hospital was 197 men, but the climate was healthy and most of the time there was little need for a hospital. On the other hand, even in the most healthful climate some people get sick. Fevers imported from outside of the Great Basin were a common ailment and violent injuries were a close second. As at some other nineteenth-century military bases, scurvy was an episodic problem at Harney. Nineteen cases appeared in 1868. An important contributing cause was the destruction of the hospital garden two years in a row by frost, grasshoppers and crickets.[25]

Built of logs with mud plastered in the cracks, the hospital was 43 feet by 34 feet and contained eight beds with 682 cubic feet of air per bed. The inside of the rooms were wainscoted. At the rear was a kitchen and mess connected to the hospital by a "rough boarded space." The ceilings of the structure were ten feet high and there were rooms for the steward, the dispensary, and a thirty by sixteen ward.[26] Also on the rear of the hospital was the wash room with two tubs and a subterranean drain. The privy serving the hospital was fifty feet behind the building.

Fort Rawlins

Fort Rawlins, like Douglas and Crittenden, was established on the eastern side of the Great Basin in Utah. Construction started on July 30, 1870, but it fulfilled the Army's need for less than a year.

------

[24]The original name honored General Frederick Steele, Columbia Department commander in 1866. General Steele changed the name to Fort Harney.

[25]*Circular No. 4.*, pp. 437-438.   [26]*Circular No 8.*, p. 467.

FORT CAMERON

As an aftermath of the Ute Black Hawk War of 1865-1868 and as a result of the "Mormon problem"—concern about the perpetrators of the Mountain Meadows massacre not being brought to justice—Fort Beaver Canyon, the last Great Basin fort to be built, was established on the Beaver River in 1872.[27] Two years later its name was changed to Fort Cameron in memory of Colonel James Cameron, killed during the Civil War battle of Bull Run.

The hospital was constructed northeast of the parade grounds. During construction, an early surgeon at the post deemed the ventilation of the ward adequate without the need of an "expensive" fireplace. The hospital, a two-story twelve-bed plastered structure, was constructed of black basaltic lava from a nearby mountain.[28] (Another account stated it was constructed of adobe with eighteen inch walls.) In November 1874 Assistant Surgeon William M. Notson noted that there was no one sick at the base and no one in the hospital.

---

[27]In 1857 a group of Mormons and their Indian allies slaughtered an emigrant party camped at Mountain Meadows in what is now the southwestern corner of Utah, in the present county of Washington, near the town of Pinto. Dunn, *Massacres of the Mountains*, pp. 237-83.

[28]Alexander and Arrington, "The Utah Military Frontier, 1872-1912, Forts Cameron, Thornburgh, and Duchesne," p. 335.

Closure of the Great Basin Forts
1866-1893

Forts McGarry, Ruby, and Churchill

Many changes in the West and on the frontier brought about the closure of the military garrisons in the Great Basin—the completion of the Central Pacific Railroad with the transcontinental telegraph, the demise of the emigrant wagon trains and the Overland Mail, the surge of the population with organized state and local militia, and the decrease in Indian hostilities. Fort McGarry closed in December 1868 and was given to peaceful Indians to be used as a reservation—Summit Lake Indian Reservation. Ten months later, in September 1869, Fort Ruby was abandoned and became the property of a private ranch.[1]

Fort Churchill was abandoned by the Army on September 29, 1869. Hostile activity in the area had ceased as a result of over sixteen thousand inhabitants living in nearby Storey County. These new inhabitants of western Nevada vastly outnumbered the Native Indians.[2] The buildings of the fort were neglected and vandalized until efforts at restoration were made in 1935. In 1957 the ruins of the fort became a Nevada historical landmark and state park, and four years later they were designated a National Historic Landmark. Located at the corner of the parade grounds the foundation

---

[1] The property is now known as Andy's Fort Ruby Ranch.

[2] Frazer, *Forts of the West*, p. 92. Also see BeDunnah, "A History of the Chinese in Nevada, 1855-1904 : A Thesis," p. 100. In 1870 there were 38,922 white inhabitants in Nevada compared to an Indian population of less than 1,000.

and portions of the wall of the hospital remain.[3] Today, sagebrush has reclaimed the parade grounds and vegetation is
growing inside the hospital ruins. Only wind can be heard
where troops once trained and Southern sympathizers
labored under armed guard.

FORTS THREE FORKS OF THE OWYHEE, SCOTT, AND RAWLINS

Three Great Basin forts—Three Forks of the Owyhee,
Scott, and Rawlins—closed in 1871 after John Shaw Billings
report, *Circular No. 4, A Report on Barracks and Hospitals with
Descriptions of Military Posts* described the condition of various military hospitals throughout the country. In the 1870
report the hospital at Fort Scott was noted by Acting Assistant Surgeons John C. Watkins and Denicke to be a sod
structure forty by twenty-four feet, with a fifteen by twenty
by nine foot ward for six patients. Continuing, the report
noted: "The building is totally unfit for a hospital."[4] Replace-
ment was not necessary since the camp closed in February
1871. One commissioned army medical officer and four
civilian doctors had served at the fort hospital.

One side of the old hospital foundation remains in 1994. It
is one hundred feet from the old adobe officer's quarters
which is now used as a private residence on a working ranch.
The foundation coincides with the location of the hospital
on the site plan and is similar to the foundation of the original hospital at Halleck. It consists of large subterranean rocks
in a pattern two feet wide.[5]

---

[3]The ruins were neglected and deteriorating when the Civilian Conservation Corps
(CCC), a welfare program during the Great Depression undertook restoration. In 1935 and
'36 several hundred men made adobe brick, rebuilt some of the adobe walls preserving the
antique appearance, and stabilized others. Their efforts are described by Housley, "Notes
and Documents: Elwood Decker and the CCC at Fort Churchill," pp. 105-21.

[4]*Circular No. 4,* p. 454.

[5]The foundation of the hospital was discovered and measured by Susan Miller Kerns,
Davey Kerns, Roy Hogan, Owen Bolstad, and Anton Sohn on November 3, 1993.

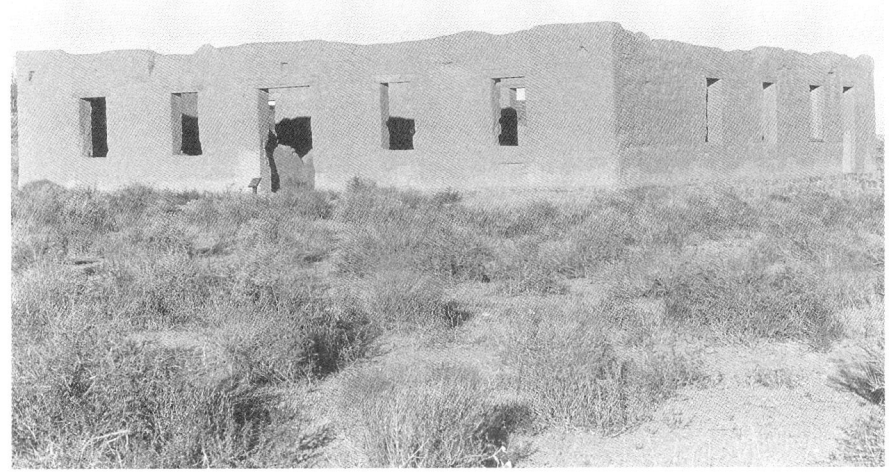

The ruins of the hospital at Fort Churchill
Photography by the author

Three Forks was abandoned and sold for $50 in 1871 without correcting the hospital's defects. No mention of the base is made in Billing's report.[6] A few months later on July 9, 1871, Fort Rawlins was abandoned. No records of its hospital were found and only one physician, Assistant Surgeon Alfred D. Wilson, served at the base.

FORTS WARNER, HARNEY, AND CAMERON

Camp Warner closed in 1874 and the command was moved to nearby Fort Harney. Also in 1874, Surgeon John E. Summers inspected Fort Cameron's hospital and found poor records and the hospital in bad repair. Six years later with the Indian threat eliminated in southeastern Oregon, the Army abandoned Fort Harney. Likewise, in Utah hostilities were subsiding. ". . . [O]n the morning of May 1st 1883 the Post

---

[6]National Archives, RG 94, E 561, pp. 429-30.

[Cameron] was abandoned" on orders from Secretary of War Robert Todd Lincoln.[7]

FORT INDEPENDENCE

Fort Independence's hospital was sold in 1883, but to regress a few years, in the spring of 1872 an earthquake destroyed the hospital and most of the fort.[8] In 1875, the military built a new frame hospital. The Army located the building which was constructed inside and out of redwood, on the north side of the parade ground. The hospital, forty by thirty-four feet, had a porch eight feet wide on the front and on both ends. The ward had five beds with 787 cubic feet of air allotted to each bed.[9]

Forty feet to the rear of the post hospital was a second building containing a fourteen by sixteen foot dead room and a fourteen by eight privy. When the fort was abandoned in July 1877, Assistant Surgeon Washington Matthews had twelve to fifteen private patients in the county hospital.[10] In 1883, the Army sold the hospital for $290 to H. P. Carter who moved it to the town of Independence where it remains today as a residence. The building was either torn down and the lumber used to build a new structure or it was extensively remodeled. The present residence has little resemblance to the original hospital.[11]

FORT HALLECK

John Shaw Billings found Fort Halleck's recently con-structed hospital unacceptable: there were no wash or bath

---

[7]National Archives, RG 94, E 547, B 69, p. 5; and Alexander, "The Utah Military Frontier," p. 337.

[8]Giffen, "Camp Independence—An Owens Valley Outpost," p. 138.

[9]Circular No. 8, p. 511.

[10]The Inyo Independent, July 14, 1877.

[11]Cragen, The Boys in the Sky-Blue Pants, p. 190, and information supplied by William H. Michael, Museum Director of the Eastern California Museum.

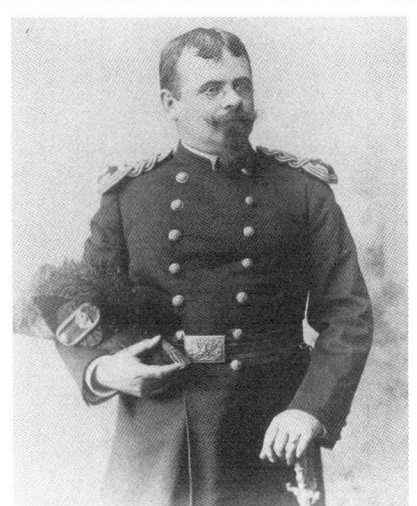

Army Doctor
Adrian Suydam Polhemus
Courtesy of National Library
of Medicine

facilities and the kitchen, laundry and deadhouse were not separated from the ward. In addition, the air space of 374 cubic feet per man was well below the 1,500 to 2,000 recommended by the Surgeon General's Office.[12]

To correct the deficiencies, the Surgeon General gave authority to build a new hospital, but a "regulation 24-bed hospital that replaced a provisional structure" was not completed until October 8, 1876.[13] Located on a hill approximately five hundred feet to the north of the old hospital, the new hospital was a two story, seventy-eight feet by twenty-six feet, frame building, with well ventilated rooms and a piazza extending around the outside.

On October 31, 1886, Lieutenant Adrian Suydam Polhemus, the twenty-seventh surgeon to serve at Fort Halleck, closed the hospital when the government abandoned the

---

[12]*Circular No. 4.*, p. VIII and p. 452.
[13]National Archives, RG 94, E 547.

base which is now occupied by a private ranch.[14] Some of the buildings were torn down and others were moved to surrounding ranches. The original hospital's foundation, consisting of large stones in a pattern two feet wide and several inches above the ground, still exists. On the other hand, all that remains of the new hospital are several foundation stones and ashes from a recent fire of another structure built on the site.[15] Today, horses wander in and out of the foundation ruins.

FORT MCDERMIT

In 1874 Acting Assistant Surgeon Kober passed through Winnemucca on assignment to Fort McDermit. He described the "best hotel" in the frontier town as "a veritable den of thugs or a bedlam of drunken cow-boys, sheep-herders, miners and prospectors, all of whom as I learned afterwards could behave decently, as long as they kept away from king alcohol."[16] In 1876 Kober heeded the criticism of Fort McDermit's hospital in the 1870 report and supervised construction of a new hospital. He carefully described it in his autobiography:

> The plan of the hospital is a slight modification of that proposed for a provisionary hospital in Circular No. 2, S.G.O., 1871. The building is one story in height, ... 43 x 38 feet, [with] a ward 24 x 24 feet ... The frame rests upon wooden piers 8 by 8 inches ... All the rooms are well lighted, and will be heated by wood stoves . . . The ward with its six windows and three transoms is especially well lighted ... The hospital is 50 yards remote from water, but barrels and buckets filled with water are kept on hand . . . The ward is painted pale green ... The isolation ward is painted blue ... a veranda on the south side of the main building . . . The striking feature of

---

[14]Ibid.

[15]On October 31, 1993, Bob Pearce, Dr. Tom Hood, Sheldon Homer, Paul Sawyer, Dick Immenschuh, Roy Hogan, Dr. Owen Bolstad, and Dr. Anton Sohn located the foundation of the old hospital and the burnt ruins near the site of the new hospital.

[16]Kober, *Reminiscences*, p. 236.

the building is that it is almost entirely constructed of lumber ...
The building ... costs only $2,216.06 in United States coin ...[17]

_____

[17]Kober, *Reminiscences*, p. 272-274. The complete description is:

The building is admirably located on a gentle slope northeast of the post, 150 yards remote from any building, and faces south by southeast. The plan of the hospital is a slight modification of that proposed for a provisionary hospital in Circular No. 2, S.G.O., 1871. The building is one story in height, and consists of an administration building 43 by 38 feet, a ward 24 by 24 feet, with an earth closet attached 8 by 10 feet. The frame rests upon wooden piers 8 by 8 inches and the space between the ground and floor of the building increases from one foot to two and a half feet in height, thus permitting of a free circulation of air beneath. The lumber and material used in the construction of the building was obtained from Truckee in the Sierra Nevada, and is of excellent quality. The exterior is lined with what is called rustic siding seven-eighths of an inch thick, dressed, and has received two coats of paint of a cream color. The flooring is five inches wide, one inch thick, tongued and grooved. For the ceiling and interior walls, sugar pine lumber, four inches wide and seven-eighths of an inch thick, dressed, tongued and grooved, has been used. The doors and transoms are all of the size described in Circular No. 2. The windows are double hung supplied with pulleys, window weights, and locks and have each twelve lights 14 by 12 inches. The roof is shingled of more than one-third pitch, and is finished with a box cornice. A ridge ventilator ten feet in length over both the ward and administration building, and a flag staff and a vane, improves the aspect of the building materially. The main building has a hall eight feet wide throughout its length; the arrangement of the rooms and their designation will be seen from the accompanying sketch. All of the rooms are well lighted, and will be heated by wood stoves; they are all twelve feet in the clear. The ward with its six windows and three transoms is especially well lighted. The arrangements for the ventilation of this room are a register one foot in diameter in the center of the floor, for the admission of pure air conducted through a "cold air box" from the exterior; a register of the same size is placed in the ceiling above for the egress of the objectionable air, and ridge ventilator completes this system of ventilation. This, together with the many doors and window, will prove sufficient means to attain thorough ventilation. A trap door 6 by 3 feet in the ceiling of the hall, the ridge ventilator, and the many windows and transoms will afford sufficient ventilation for the administration building. The kitchen is a frame building 14 by 14 feet and was moved from the old hospital to its present position twelve feet in rear of the dining room. It was considered prudent to have this building disconnected. The hospital is 50 yards remote from water, but barrels and buckets filled with water are kept on hand. The dispensary is supplied with a neat medicine case, counter, and drawers and is complete in all its appointments. The storeroom had been well supplied with shelves and two coats of paint. Instead of a pure white color, some pigments have been added, which are quite pleasing to the eye. The ward is painted pale green derived from an admixture of Prussian blue and chrome yellow; the halls and other rooms are painted with the same color. The isolation ward is painted blue, the windows of this apartment are stained blue, and the whole affords a light most soothing to the eye and likely to be specially adapted for cases of delirium tremens and the delirium of low fevers. The additions recently authorized, consisting of a veranda on the south side of the main building, an enclosure around the hospital, and erection of a woodshed, have not been completed. Some of the material is now being hauled to the post. After the veranda is competed it is proposed to close up the sides between the floors of the piazza and the ground with lattice work. All the work on the building has been well done, and,

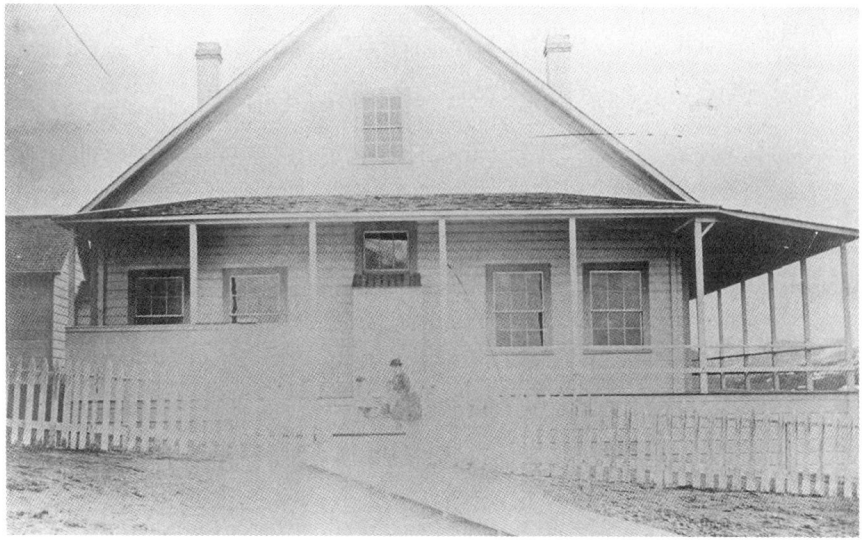

The hospital at Fort McDermit
Courtesy of Judy and Fred Wilkinson

A picture of the hospital taken in 1880 shows a porch surrounding the structure and large windows providing the necessary ventilation. Today, nothing remains of the new hospital. As with other abandoned Great Basin forts the

though it is called Provisionary Hospital, it is complete in all its appointments and likely to be of great durability. The striking feature of the building is that it is almost entirely constructed of lumber. This was a measure of economy as the material requested for plastering could only be obtained eighty miles from the post, and because the work itself would have entailed a considerable outlay. As it was, the carpenter completed the whole building (painting excepted) for $400, a greater amount would have been necessary for the plastering work alone. In a hygienic point of view, I consider the present walls of the hospital less liable to absorb noxious gases and disease germ than other hard finished walls and an occasional coat of paint will render them still more impervious. In case of necessity, much of the material used in the construction of a building of this kind, the ceiling lumber included, could be taken down and used elsewhere. The painting and the construction for the chimneys was done by enlisted men, and all the material was hauled from Winnemucca, eighty-four miles distant, by the post transportation. The building, which costs only $2,216.06 in United States coin, is a credit to the commanding officer and post quartermaster, who have added their might to render the construction a complete success.

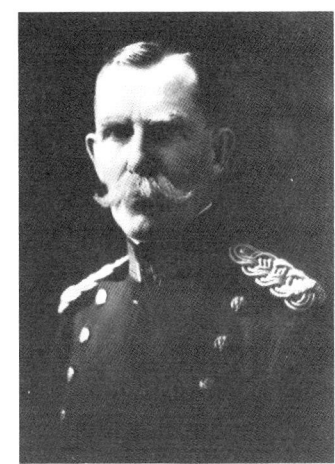

Army Doctor
William Pratt Kendall
Courtesy of National Library
of Medicine

lumber and buildings were removed and used for other purposes. However, the legacy of Indian health care remains and a modern clinic staffed by United States Public Health personnel rests near the site of Kober's hospital.

Equipment in the 1876 hospital included a Beck's binocular microscope and a chest of chemicals to test water and urine. Dr. Kober also described the library as a "very good hospital library with the best texts and copies of the *American Journal of Medical Science, London Lancet, British Medical Journal* and the *New York Medical Record*."[18] For transportation, Dr. Kober had horses and a Daugherty spring wagon that was also used as an ambulance and for transportation.

Kober and Corbusier were the most notable physicians who rotated through the command but seventeen other doctors served at the hospital. Dr. William Pratt Kendall, the last surgeon to serve in a nineteenth-century Nevada military post, closed the hospital on June 15, 1889, and signed the hospital ledger:

----

[18]Ibid., p. 268.

No patients admitted, no births, marriages or death . . . No meteorological observations made from [the] 1st . . . Weather had been
very dry and warm: water already becoming scarce in the Quin
[Quinn] River and adjacent valleys.[19]

Meteorological observations were taken by Army doctors
because of the notion that climate and weather affected
health. When Kendall signed the ledger in 1889 the bacterial
cause of disease was gaining acceptance by many physicians
and as a result the role of climate and weather on health was
being modified. The germ theory had started a profound
revolution in medicine that would last through the twentieth
century.

FORT BIDWELL

*Circular No. 8, A report on the Hygiene of the United States
Army with Descriptions of Military Posts* in 1875 found further
problems with poorly constructed hospitals and authority
was given to build a new Fort Bidwell hospital. The old hospital was "badly arranged and decayed." Moreover, Assistant
Surgeons Daniel G. Caldwell and Charles Smart found the
rooms unlined and "uncomfortably cold" in the winter.

In 1875 the Army erected a new hospital, a "modern"
frame building with a twelve-patient ward, isolation room,
bathroom, dispensary, office, store room, kitchen, mess-
room, steward's quarters, cook's quarters, nurse's quarters
and mortuary.[20] The surgeon located the hospital on a slope,
today known as Hospital Hill, eight hundred feet from the
officers' quarters. A fire destroyed the building in 1928 and
on the site a new hospital and tuberculosis sanitarium for
Native Indians was built.[21]

The sanitarium is now in ruins and the only building

---

[19]National Archives, RG 94 , E 547 and 561.
[20]*Circular No. 8,* p. 502.
[21]George Martin Kober Manuscript.

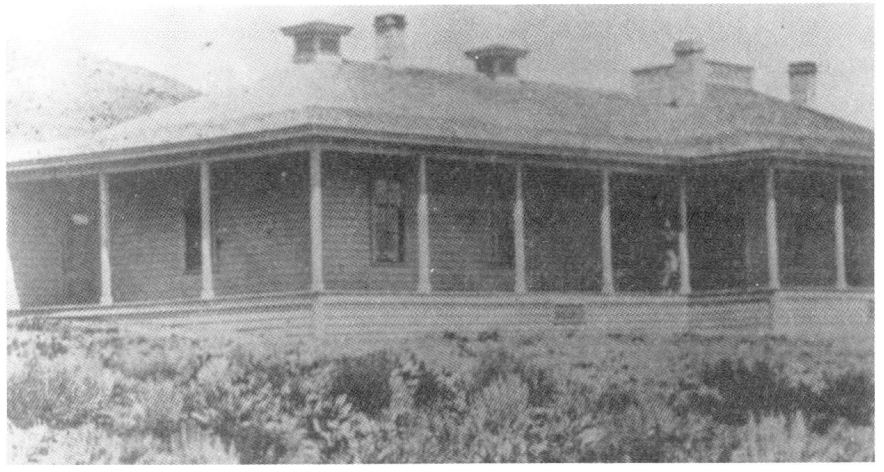

Fort Bidwell Hospital, 1870s
Courtesy of Patricia A. Barry

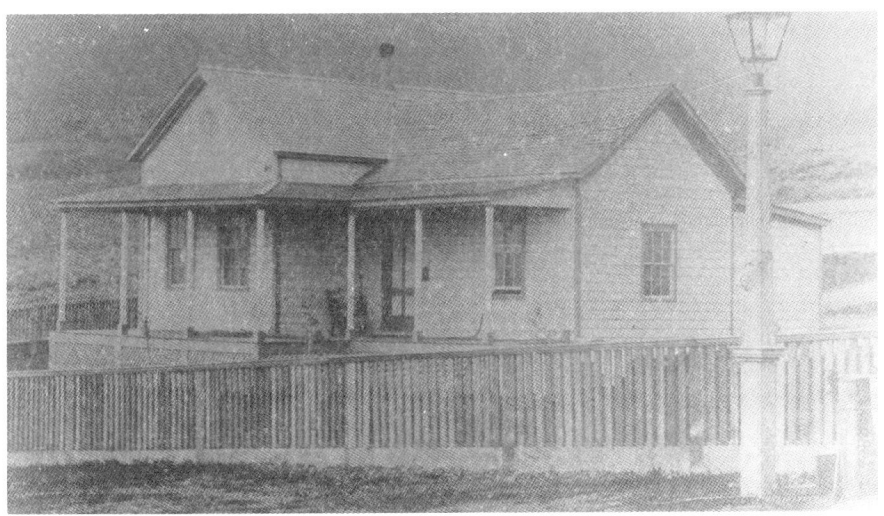

Kober's Quarters at Fort Bidwell, 1885
Courtesy of Patricia A. Barry

remaining from the halcyon days of the fort is the decaying school/chapel on the northeast corner of the parade grounds. There are nineteen military graves in the nearby cemetery, including one for a soldier from Fort Warner, dating from the military period. The original cemetery is still used by citizens of the community.

As a result of the decreased hostilities and the growth of the civilian population the Army abandoned the post in 1893. In 1897, Congress gave authority to the Department of Interior to convert Fort Bidwell into an Indian school. The fort buildings were used to construct the school and homes.

FORT DOUGLAS

Changes were also necessary over the years at Fort Douglas to meet military code and modern ideas of hospital construction. A kitchen and post-mortem room were added, and a new hospital was built in 1875 to accommodate the demands of the fort. Orders stated that the cost was not to exceed $9,000. Description of the new hospital, built between April 26, 1875, and September 1, 1875, consisted of a two story main building, thirty by eighty-four feet and a one story brick addition, twenty-four by sixty feet.[22]

---

[22] A description of the hospital is found in RG 77 at the National Archives. A copy of the description is also in the Fort Douglas Museum, Salt Lake City. A 1½ page condensation of the 23 page description follows:

Construction authorized by the Honorable Secretary of War.
April 12th 1875

The drawings herewith have been prepared with exactness and show clearly the several elevations, plans, sections and details of construction.

The Hospital is designed for 16 patients, but a greater number could be accommodated in case of emergency.

General Description

The building is 83' 4" long, 29' 4" wide and two stories high, the lower story 12' and the upper 15' in the clear. A piazza also two stories high, extends entirely around. The material used in exterior walls & foundation is a light red sand stone which was obtained on the military reservation. The stone is hard and quartzitic, but works freely under the chisel. It is quite porous, absorbs water freely, but does not crumble or exfoliate when exposed to the frost.

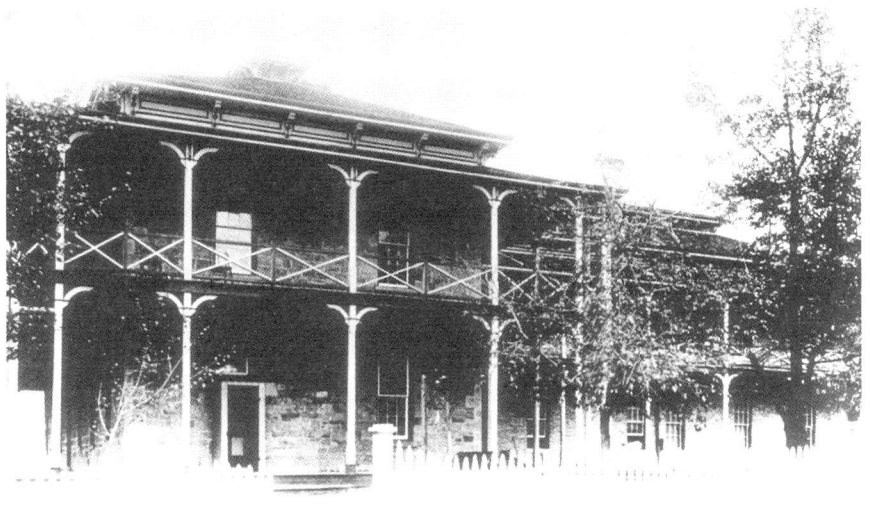

Fort Douglas Hospital, 1875
Courtesy of Fort Douglas Military Museum

By 1893 the hospital had been replaced with a stone structure with two wards and a twenty-four-bed isolation ward.
Heat was now provided by a steam heater, but adequate ventilation was still an important consideration. Ridge ventilation and fresh air inlets at the floor level were added. To
provide nutrition for the troops on duty, "Two cows and a
quantity of chickens were kept for use of the sick."[23]

The building is covered with a hip roof, surrounded by a ventilator the entire length of
the ridge, and is provided with louvered ventilating spaces. Entirely around, both on main
roof and piazza, a deck gutter, lined with tin, is formed and tin conductors lead to the
ground.

Excavations

The natural slope, on which the Hospital stands has a fall of about one foot in ten, the
grade falling off towards the south west, the soil being rather sandy loam, but containing
enough argillaceous property to compact well, and when the alluvium upon the surface was
cleared off, a good foundation to build upon was obtained. The trenches for foundation
walls were dug to the depth of 2½ feet beneath the natural surfaces, and 2½ ft. wide. The
piers to support the piazza and interior bearers of floor joists were also set 2½ feet in depth.

[23]"Fort Douglas Medical History," Fort Douglas Museum, Salt Lake City.

Assistant Surgeon William Hemple Arthur recalled the stone building:

> There was a 40-bed stone hospital with some modern improvements, but even here the building was very primitive. There was no laboratory or operating room, no running water except from a hydrant outside of the kitchen, no water closets. It was considered the finest military hospital in the Department of the Platte, if not in all the west.[24]

During Arthur's tenure (1883-1886) at Fort Douglas, the only professional challenge was a "serious outbreak of typhoid fever." Like other frontier surgeons, he was in charge of the hospital garden, a two and one half acre plot.[25]

This overview of some of the doctors and military hospitals in the Great Basin raises questions about the quality of health care and the health of troops stationed in the area. If the hospitals did not meet the sanitary standards of the time, what about the general sanitary conditions at the forts? If the training of some of the doctors was inadequate, did the men, on the whole, receive good treatment? How available were wholesome food and medicine, and how were medical emergencies handled? Since health care in the territory was embryonic, were civilians and Native Indians deprived of vital supplies and services that were available to the Army. How did the health of civilians and the Native Indians care compare to that of military personnel? What diseases were prevalent in the military, in the civilian population, and among the Native Indians?

In order to answer these questions it is necessary to look at education and licensing of nineteenth-century physicians, knowledge of disease, medical supplies, duties and responsibilities of the surgeons, assisting personnel, and the doctors' position in the army.

---

[24] Ashburn, *A History of the Medical Department of the United States Army*, p. 118.
[25] *Circular No. 4*, p. 364.

Physician Training and Knowledge of Disease in the Late-Nineteenth Century

PHYSICIAN TRAINING[1]

In the mid-nineteenth century the quality of medical education in the United States was generally considered to be poor. Before the Civil War, no medical college in the United States compared with the best European schools.[2] One method of obtaining medical training was to pay $100 a year for an apprenticeship with a practicing physician, or a student took didactic courses consisting of two, repetitive, non-graded, four-month courses. Some students combined both methods of training while others attended and graduated from several medical colleges in order to get more experience. Even so, well into the nineteenth century some medical students learned their craft outside of conventional medical systems and had little undergraduate teaching or medical education.[3]

Like other American medical colleges, Dr. Elias Samuel Cooper's school in San Francisco, the first medical school in California, required two repetitive eighteen-week terms with

---

[1]Some of this information is published in Sohn, "19th-Century Academic Examinations for Physicians in the United States Army Medical Department," pp. 472-74.

[2]O'Malley, *The History of Medical Education*.

[3]Martin Kaufman, "American Medical Education," in Ronald L. Numbers, ed., *The Education of American Physicians*, p. 7.

one of the terms being in San Francisco.[4] But when established in 1858, Cooper Medical College (later, Stanford University Medical School) was more progressive than many schools and had a prerequisite of a one year apprenticeship under a respected physician or a high school diploma.

In 1871, the Chicago Medical College alone provided a top quality medical education with a five month graded course and a prerequisite of a college education or an admission examination.[5] Most medical schools required no prerequisites—proficiency in reading and writing, or mental or physical fitness.[6] In addition, no accrediting body assured the quality of the curriculum or inspected medical schools thereby allowing diploma mills to proliferate during the 1870s and '80s. In fact, in today's climate of regulation, all nineteenth-century medical schools would be considered diploma mills.

In 1850, one area of the country, eastern Tennessee, only 35 of 201 doctors had graduated from a regular medical school.[7] The situation in East Tennessee may not have been representative of the country as a whole, but it demonstrated the inconsistency in medical education in the mid-nineteenth century. By the end of the century medical education was improving, but it left much to be desired.

Records show that 608 doctors either practiced medicine

---

[4]Harris, *California's Medical Story*, Dr. Elias Samuel Cooper organized the first medical school in California in 1858 by obtaining a charter from the University of the Pacific, a Methodist school in San Jose. Cooper's school was chartered as the Medical Department of the University of the Pacific, pp. 131-134. The Medical College of the Pacific (reorganized as a Presbyterian College) became Cooper Medical College in 1882. In 1912 it became Stanford Medical School, p. 139.

[5]Kaufman, "American Medical Education," in Numbers, ed., *The Education of American Physicians,* pp. 14-15.

[6]See Shryock, *Medical Licensing in America, 1650-1965*, for a discussion of medical licensing in the nineteenth century.

[7]See Rothstein, *American Physicians in the Nineteenth Century*, for a discussion of medical education in the nineteenth century.

in Nevada or came to the state between 1855 and 1900.[8] Included are twenty-three women, all of whom were noted after 1864. Records stating the school of graduation were located on 46 percent (281 physicians) for the forty-five-year period.[9] Most (203 or 72.2%) were American graduates from a regular medical college, 26 (9.3%) graduated from a foreign medical school, 36 (12.8%) graduated from an eclectic school, fourteen (5.0%) graduated from a homeopathic school, and two (0.7%) graduated from a school of unknown philosophy.[10] Even though 9.3 percent were foreign graduates, 25.4 percent (65 of 256 on whom the place of birth was recorded) were foreign born, reflecting the intense immigration of the nineteenth century.

Not only was medical education uncontrolled and inconsistent during most of the nineteenth century, but medical regulation was also at a low level. After 1830 state legislatures were reluctant to control the profession. Indeed, between 1830 and 1860 Jacksonian philosophy engulfed the citizens of the young democracy where "Freedom of choice" became more important than protection of the public from unscrupulous and quack medical practitioners.

One widely read author in 1840, Dr. John C. Gunn, asserted that practically every aspect of medicine could be practiced by unskilled individuals. In his *Domestic Medicine* the medical practice was reduced to "common sense" and was proposed "for families of Western and Southern States."[11]

---

[8]The total does not include a complete review of newspaper advertisements from the nineteenth century. The statistics may be weighted toward legitimate physicians who might be more inclined to state their school of graduation. The newspapers at that time carried many advertisements for Dr. XYZ and his amazing machine or cure-all or all-healing medicine.

[9]Incomplete records are due to loss of records from fires and inconsistent recording practices.

[10]Irregular schools taught botanical and the herbal treatment of disease.

[11]Rosenberg, *Explaining Epidemics*, pp. 57 and 62.

Since many states did not require a medical license, any-one could hang out a sign or shingle proclaiming a title and a willingness to treat patients. State lobbyists successfully promoted this philosophy and allowed Thomsoniasm, a botanical medical sect, and other unorthodox medical groups such as eclectics and homeopaths to thrive and practice without controls. It was said by a pretentious European that, "in no country in the world is quackery carried on to so enormous an extent as it is in the United States . . . thus it is no uncommon thing to find a person calling himself a Doctor in New York . . . up to the very day that he left for 'the land of liberty,' had been . . . a shoe maker, tailor or liquor dealer."[12] However, fifty years later the problem was restated by an American, Abraham Flexner.

> We have indeed in America medical practitioners not inferior to the best elsewhere; but here is probably no other country in the world in which there is so great a distance and so fatal a difference between the best, the average, and the worst.[13]

It was noted in California during the early 1850s that the title of doctor was given "to anyone who practices medicine or who desires to be so called."[14] Furthermore, the Supreme Court of Michigan made a ruling that remained in effect until 1883 stating that, "A doctor is any person calling himself such."[15]

A French visitor to the United States noted that of the eight "doctors" in Monterey, California, in 1851 only two were full-time practitioners worthy of the title, "physician." Three were merchants who sold medicine along with other wares, two were farmers and the last pulled teeth and operated a combination drug and novelty store.

---

[12]Prendergast, "Quackery and the Quacked," pp. 354-59.

[13]Flexner, *Medical Education in the United States and Canada*, p. 20.

[14]Garnier, *A Medical Journey in California*, pp. 64-65.

[15]Ackerknecht, *Malaria in the Upper Mississippi Valley, 1760-1900*, p. 11.

In San Jose, an Italian wig-maker practiced as a doctor and pharmacist.[16] This state of affairs extended across the Great Basin where many tradesmen usurped the position of doctor, dentist or pharmacist in their adopted town. By simply hanging out a sign advertising a drugstore or pharmacy, the proprietor could deceive the public and practice the healing arts while selling "snake oil."

In the 1870s in Nevada, Dr. Henry Bergstein was elected to the Nevada Assembly with the stated purpose of enacting legislation to require the registration of medical licenses. He was appalled by a druggist in Bullionville who practiced medicine to the detriment of the local miners. Bergstein wrote:

> One of the most prominent symptoms of lead colic is an obstinate constipation, and in a number of cases which applied to him [the druggist] for relief, he ran the gamut of cathartics from salts to croton oil; all failing him, he gave liquid quicksilver, and succeeded only in giving them a passage to the grave.[17]

These unscientific practices also concerned the United States Army and its applicants for the medical examination. The Army was only interested in having regular physicians in its Medical Department. As a result some applicants emphatically stated that they had never practiced homeopathy. If a homeopathic doctor wished to practice medicine in the military he had to deny his homeopathic background. For example, a homeopathic physician practicing in Maine in 1864 passed himself off as a regular physician in order to get an appointment in the Union army as a military surgeon.[18]

Homeopaths treated disease with minute doses of drugs which produce the same symptom as exhibited by the illness.

---

[16]Gamier, *A Medical Journey in California*, pp. 65-67.

[17]Davis, ed., *The History of Nevada*, v. I, p. 611.

[18]Warner, *The Therapeutic Prospective*, p. 181.

In contrast to homeopathy, allopathy or regular medicine was defined as a system of treatment that seeks to cure a disease by alleviating the symptom produced by the disease. Considering some of the harsh and severe therapeutics used by regular doctors in the nineteenth century, homeopathic drug therapy was a viable option, even though it was founded on unscientific principles. As a consequence, homeopathy and other alternative treatments thrived.

By 1850 only New Jersey and the District of Columbia had licensing laws controlling medical practice. In 1854 New Jersey eliminated its controls.[19] At the start of the Civil War there was minimal regulation of medical practice. Slowly, states began regulation, and by the end of 1881 one half of the states and territories had some degree of licensure.[20] By 1893, eighteen states required an examination and seventeen other states required a medical school diploma.[21] Nevada required local registration and a diploma in 1875, but a doctor with ten years practice was exempt. Not until 1899 did Nevada legislate and enforce state-wide licensure.

Civilian practice aside, the army confronted the problem and established strict academic examinations for successful medical officer candidates. The high education and fitness standards of the U. S. Army and Navy medical corps were recognized by the various states and territories, exempting them from local examination. As late as 1897 it was said that, "The common soldiers and enlisted sailors are the only classes of the population of this great country protected, by law and regulation alike, from incompetent medical service and a mercenary pharmacy."[22] Even with high military standards,

---

[19]See Ramsey, "The Politics of Professional Monopoly in Nineteenth Century Medicine," pp. 225-306, and Shryock, *Medical Licensing in America, 1650-1965.*

[20]Baker, "Physician Licensure Laws in the United States, 1865-1915," p. 174.

[21]Rosen, *The Structure of American Medical Practice,* p. 20.

[22]Busey, "The Organization, High *Esprit De Corps,* High Standard of Education and Scientific Attainments of the Army Medical Department," pp. 6-7.

civilian doctors who were substandard received military contracts at post hospitals. However, once the contract was signed, scrutiny continued and the Army annulled contracts when the individual performed poorly.

KNOWLEDGE OF DISEASE IN THE NINETEENTH CENTURY

In 1814 Surgeon-General James Tilton required all army doctors to keep meteorological, climatic and wind data.[23] The theory then, was that miasmas resulting from foul air, pollution, and vapors due to decomposition of vegetable and animal matter from marshes and along rivers caused disease.[24] Surgeon General Joseph Lovell in 1818 wrote:

> Every physician who makes a science of his profession or arrives at eminence in it will keep a journal of this nature, as the influence of weather and climate upon diseases, especially epidemics, is well known. From the circumstances of the soldier, their effects upon diseases of the army are peculiarly interesting, as by proper management they may in a great measure be obviated, To this end every surgeon should be furnished with a good thermometer, and, in addition to a diary of the weather should note everything relative to the topography of his station, the climate, complaints prevalent in the vicinity, etc., that may tend to discover the causes of diseases, to the promotion of health, and the improvement of medical science.[25]

Lovell's main concern was to understand the weather and climate as related to the cause of disease and epidemics. If one could control environmental factors such as "complaints prevalent in the vicinity" and foul vapors, the transmission of disease could be better controlled. Modifications of the miasma theory persisted through the end of the nineteenth century.

The foul vapor theory had wide support. At the fourth

---

[23]Ibid., p. 7.
[24]Coffman, *The Old Army*, pp. 182-84.
[25]Kober, *Reminiscences*, p.149.

National Quarantine and Sanitary Convention in 1859-1860, miasmas and gases were regarded as important in transmission of disease. In addition poisons in the environment were considered a cause of disease. Cholera, an important infectious disease of the nineteenth century, in the mid-century was believed to be caused by a specific organic poison.[26]

Also, "earthy matter" in the drinking water was a cause for diarrhea and disease. (See Corson's army medical examination, pages 110-11 below.) Kober stated in his report of August 1875 from Fort McDermit that decomposition of vegetation polluted the base's water supply and was the cause of the high incidence of disease.[27] Assistant Surgeon Charles B. Byrne earlier in April 1872 reported that the water supply was the cause of illness at Fort Warner.[28] A report from Fort Douglas in April 1872 left no question how illness was spread. "Officer's families were sick more often than laundresses and their families. This was undoubtedly due to the fact that laundresses quarters were situated along Red Butte Creek and above the main post where officers lived."[29]

In August 1883 eight cases of typhoid were in the Fort Douglas hospital. A Special Sanitary report recommended that:

> . . . some rapid method be at once adopted to clean out the reservoir (an open pond east of the post) from which drinking water of the post is obtained, and the larger sewer from which drinking water of the post is obtained, and the larger sewer drain be flushed by fresh water every other day.[30]

In addition to water, food was often considered to be a

---

[26]Richmond, "American Attitudes Toward the Germ Theory of Disease," pp. 58 and 59.

[27]National Archives, RG 94, E 547.

[28]National Archives, RG 94, E 547, B 328.

[29]"Fort Douglas Medical History," Fort Douglas Museum, Salt Lake City.

[30]Ibid.

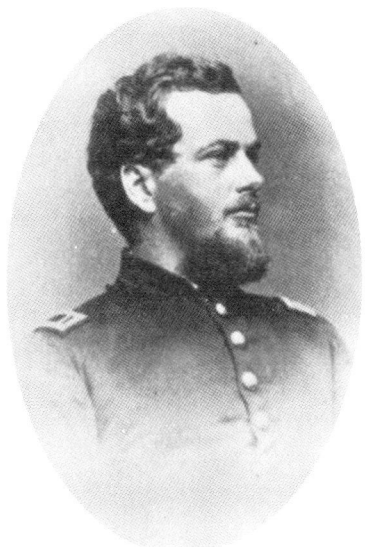

Assistant Surgeon
Charles H. Byrne
Courtesy of National Library
of Medicine

source of disease. Corbusier thought that contaminated flour used to make bread was the cause of the base's outbreak of diarrhea and fever among the Indians at Fort McDermit in July 1870.[31] For certain, dough or flour, contaminated with a virulent bacteria could cause infectious diarrhea, but the dough most likely would be sterilized in the baking process. However, bread contaminated after baking could cause illness.

Even worse for the morale of the troops was the alleged contamination of the liquor supply. In May 1878 Assistant Surgeon Washington Matthews reported "many cases of illness due to bad liquor sold in the village" [of Fort Bidwell].[32] Although illness, probably infectious, could be spread through the food supply it is unlikely that liquor would be the source.

[31]National Archives, RG 94, E 547, B 410.
[32]National Archives, RG 94, E 547, B104.

These military surgeons did not know the bacterial etiology of disease. The proof of the germ theory had to wait for
the identification of a specific organism as the cause of a specific disease, but they did understand fevers and were able to
relate certain types of fevers to an underlying cause. An
important nineteenth-century doctor, Daniel Drake, in 1850
listed fourteen fevers important to infectious diseases:

> Autumnal, bilious, intermittent, remittent, congestive, miasmatic,
> malarial, marsh, malignant, chill-fever, ague,[33] fever and ague,
> dumb ague, and lastly the Fever ... they can change from one to the
> other. An intermittent turns into remittent and assuming the for-
> mer can become first, a quotidian, then a tertian, and finally, a
> quartan.[34]

These are various forms of malaria (*mal aria* or bad air)
that refer to the time of the year, type of fever or origin from a
marsh. The cause of malaria was thought to be from bad air,
especially from decaying vegetable matter from swamps.
Cases of malaria in areas where swamps were not found led to
a resurgence of the animalcular hypothesis of disease in the
early nineteenth century.[35] Drake used the theory to explain
the different forms of malaria as caused by different species
of small insects. He stopped just short of describing the mosquito in the transmission of malaria.[36]

Hospital returns (reports to the surgeon general from base
surgeons) from the various Great Basin forts echo this concern with fevers. The hospital census of Fort Churchill for
the first eighteen months of operation listed 655 admissions,

---

[33] Ague was a British term referring to the chills associated with malaria.

[34] Drake, *A Systematic Treatise, Historical, Etiological, and Practical on the Principal Diseases of the Interior Valley of North America,* pp. 703-704. Drake (1785-1852) was leader in
Ohio and Kentucky and helped establish medical teaching in those states. He traveled
widely and published the above important two volume treatise on medicine and infectious
disease. His writings influenced medical students and practicing doctors.

[35] Ackerknecht, *Malaria in the Upper Mississippi Valley 1760-1900,* p. 12. The animalcular theory held that disease was caused by minute animals.

[36] Ibid., p. 13-14.

of which 121 (18%) were for fevers. Forts Halleck and McDermit for 1873-1874 list intermittent fever as the most common disease (20% of the diseases reported to the surgeon general) at the posts.[37]

Intermittent fever was identified as malarial fever by its alternating periods of fever and chills. Various fevers were treated with quinine, an agent widely used in nineteenth-century America and one that was effective against the malaria parasite. In contrast, some of the Paiutes had a simple approach to the treatment of infectious disease. When smallpox infected families they were eliminated by other members of the tribe without a trace. In some tribes, suicide resulted when symptoms occurred.[38]

Later, as a result of the discovery of the etiology of infectious disease, techniques in surgery improved.[39] Surgery became safer due to control of intra- and postoperative infections. In 1876, Sir Joseph Lister visited Philadelphia and emphasized antiseptic surgery. American physicians listened with interest and reluctantly introduced his suggested changes in operating technique.

In 1877 the U. S. Army took the lead and made antisepsis a requirement in surgery. Major George Miller Sternberg, a medical officer in the United States Army, was instrumental in establishing disinfection in military procedure.[40] Captain

---

[37]*Circular No. 8*, p. 511.

[38]Stone, *Medicine Among the American Indians*, p. 56.

[39]Toward the end of the military era in the Great Basin, the microbial cause of disease was described on a regular basis—anthrax in 1869, typhoid fever 1880, leprosy 1880, malaria 1880, tuberculosis 1882, cholera 1883, and diphtheria 1884. As this information and the technology of bacteria culture spread from Europe, bacteriology was included in the curriculum of American schools. Dr. T. S. Burril gave a few lectures on bacteria at the University of Illinois in the 1870s and Dr. Henry Formad included the subject in his lectures at the University of Pennsylvania in 1882. Eggerth, *The History of the Hoagland Laboratory*, p. 12

[40]Eggerth, *The History of the Hoagland Laboratory*, p. 11. Sternberg became Surgeon General of the Army (1883-92). He also was the first person in the United States to demonstrate the organisms of malaria (1885) and tuberculosis and typhoid (1886). Phalen, *Chiefs of the Medical Department United States Army*, pp. 72-73.

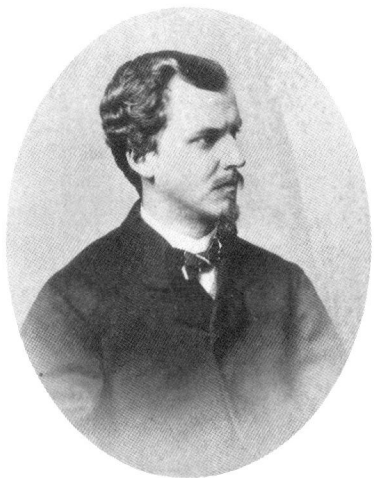

Army Doctor Alfred C. Girard
Courtesy of National Library of Medicine

Alfred C. Girard, in *Circular Orders No. 3,* published Lister's system of antiseptic surgery using carbolized dressings, carbolized sutures and sprays.[41] Yet, as late as 1878 antisepsis was not universally used or accepted in this country.[42]

These prevailing philosophies of disease made Surgeon Kober's treatment at Fort McDermit of an infected shotgun injury in 1874 an innovative act. Edward McMorrow went hunting in December 1874 and left his gun in the bushes. He returned the next day and picked up the gun by the barrel. It accidentally discharged wounding him in the hand and knee. When his horse returned to the base alone, a party of men and Kober went out to search for him. After returning to base with the wounded soldier, Kober applied alcohol and carbolic acid to the wounds and amputated the finger. For anesthesia, Kober prescribed two ounces of whiskey.

On January 9, pus formation became evident in the knee

---

[41]Captain Girard later served from 1895-1898 at Fort Douglas.
[42]Cozen, "Military Orthopedic Surgery," p. 52. Also, see Bayne-Jones, *The Evolution of Preventive Medicine in the United States Army,* pp. 115-16.

wound. On the 21st, Kober proposed amputation and McMorrow's refusal propelled George Martin Kober's treatment into medical history. On January 28, he started injections of the wound with tincture of iodine, carbolic acid and glycerin. This was the first treatment on record of an infection using this technique.[43] The knee wound healed on June 28 when the last abscess sealed over.

By 1882, the proper treatment of a wound required irrigation with water, application of corrosive sublimate solution, dusting of iodoform powder into the wound and application of an antiseptic dressing.[44] The use of the thermometer also helped to diagnose and control infections.[45]

The bacterial cause of disease became accepted, but the influence of climate on disease was still important. In a paper presented to the Texas State Medical Association in 1895, Dr. I. M. Cline stated:

> The air breathed, its temperature, vapor of water, purity and pressure, the amount of sunshine received, the character of the winds, and the nature of the soil, all have a potent influence upon the organism in health in causing or preventing disease; and a still more potent influence upon it in its unstable and sensitive condition when already the subject of disease.[46]

Cline studied over 125 diseases and concluded that mortality was related to increases or decreases of daily temperatures. Furthermore, sudden changes in the weather were unfavorable to the successful treatment of most diseases. A precipitous drop in temperature was most harmful.[47]

---

[43]Kober, "Report of a Case of Gunshot Wound of the Right Knee Joint and Right Hand," pp. 427-33. Kober's treatment is also mentioned in the footnotes of *The Medical and Surgical History of the Civil War, Part III. v. II. Surgical History,* p. 418.

[44]Cozen, "Military Orthopedic Surgery," p. 52.

[45]Garrison, *Notes on the History of Military Medicine,* p. 181.

[46]Cline, "The Climatic Causation of Disease," p. 2. This theory of "epidemic constitution" dates to Thomas Sydenham in the 17th century. Bynum and Nutton, eds., *Theories of Fever from Antiquity to the Enlightenment,* p. 69.

[47]Ibid., pp. 5-6.

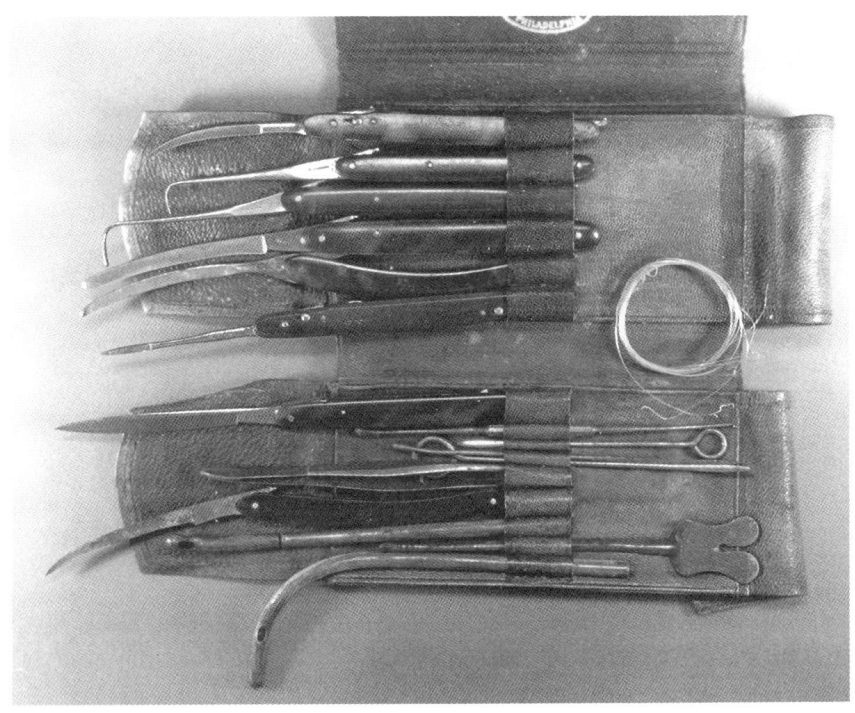

Nineteenth Century Pocket Medical Instruments
Photography by author, University of Nevada School of Medicine Collection

The Practice of Medicine at the Great Basin Military Hospitals

During the period of military presence in the Great Basin a surgeon had a limited number of instruments and drugs to use in his practice. Common instruments available included chisels, probes, gouges, mallets, several kinds of saws and an assortment of forceps.[1] Surgery consisted primarily of amputating limbs, probing wounds, and lancing abscesses.

Many surgeons were also trained to trephine the skull as Kober did at Fort McDermit. He claimed to have treated four or five patients with skull fractures by trephination without any fatalities.[2] The instruments used in these surgical procedures were sometimes provided and owned by the surgeon. When Acting Assistant Surgeon Samuel F. Chapin signed a contract in 1865 for $113 a month the Army asked him to provide amputating, trephining, and pocket instruments. The document further stated that the Army would provide the instruments if Chapin could not supply them.[3]

Other instruments such as microscopes, thermometers and testing equipment were supplied by the military. Even though a major category of disease was fevers, not until 1865 was clinical thermometry taught in the New York Hospital.

---

[1]Hunt, *The Army of the Pacific,* p. 267.

[2]Kober, *Reminiscences,* p. 271. Trephination is accomplished by drilling a small 1-1½ cm hole in the skull to remove a blood clot or release pressure.

[3]National Archives, RG 94, E 561.

In 1868, a patient thermometer was provided in the military doctor's instrument bag along with an assortment of drugs.[4]

Of the drugs supplied at the posts, chloroform and opium compounds were probably the most important. These drugs made pain bearable. However, an older remedy, whiskey, was still used as Kober did when he amputated McMorrow's finger.[5] If a patient was too weak for chloroform anesthesia, doctors prescribed liberal doses of whiskey and strychnia (strychnine), a treatment regimen used until the end of the nineteenth century.[6]

An archeological survey of the Fort Churchill in the 1970s gives some indication of the drugs used at the post. Excavation of the hospital area revealed the following bottle fragments: whiskey, gin, wine, brandy, schnapps, Champagne, Perry Davis Vegetable Pain Killer, Stomach Bitters (tonic), and cod liver oil.[7] This list might reinforce the fact that escape from the hard realities of life in the West was sought in the whiskey bottle. Even more important is what it tells us about medical therapeutics during the era.

The high concentration of alcohol containers around the Fort Churchill hospital indicates physicians encouraged the use of alcohol as a "stimulant." Champagne, brandy, and port wine also were given to patients who were weak from disease.[8] Even infants were treated with doses of alcohol. A six-months-old baby diagnosed with "Remittent fever" at Fort Warner in November 1867 was treated with quinine, beef tea and sherry wine.[9] (Quinine, Cinchona bark and iron compounds were also frequently used as stimulants by physicians in the 1860s.[10])

---

[4]Rosenberg, *Explaining Epidemics*, p. 144, and Kober, *Reminiscences*, p. 36.
[5]Kober, "Report of a Case of Gunshot Wound," pp. 427-33.
[6]Senn, *Medico-Surgical Aspects of the Spanish American War*, p. 200.
[7]Hardesty, "Historical Archaeology at Fort Churchill," p. 287.
[8]Senn, *Medico-Surgical Aspects of the Spanish American War*, p. 200.
[9]Gilliss, *So Far from Home*, p. 156.
[10]Warner, *The Therapeutic Prospective*, p. 98.

The use of alcohol was also popular in folk medicine as a home remedy. Various forms of alcohol were used in alcoholic bitters and elixirs. One of the most famous of the bitters, Hostetter's Bitters, contained 32 percent alcohol along with various herbs. Some saloons even served Hostetter's Bitters at the bar like any other alcoholic drink.

Besides alcohol other therapeutic compounds used in the West were camphor (an anti-infective and antipruritic agent), castor oil (a purgative), calomel (an antiseptic, cathartic and salivant), flaxseed oil (a demulcent), ginger (a flavoring agent), horehound (a mint used for flavoring), laudanum (a tincture containing opium), spirit of ammonia (a disinfectant), blue vitriol (an irritant, astringent and fungicide), carbolic acid (disinfectant and antiseptic), Epsom salt (laxative and local anti-inflammatory agent), hartshorn (expectorant and used in smelling salts), sulfur (used to treat rheumatism, gout, bronchitis, and externally in the treatment of skin diseases) and turpentine (for worms and topical application).[11]

A better idea of the drugs used by surgeons during the era of Nevada frontier military medicine is demonstrated by a review of the medicine available to Civil War surgeons. They carried a medical supply pannier on a horse with fifty-two medical compounds sold by Edward R. Squibb, M.D. Some of the items included in his kit were: morphine, chloroform, ipecac, colchicine (used for gout), ether, mercury pills (diuretic and purging agent), alcohol, quinine (antipyretic), Cantharides or "Spanish fly" (counter-irritant and vesicant), creosote (disinfectant), valerian (a root used as a sedative), tea, sugar, coffee, condensed milk and beef extract.[12]

This list reflects medical therapeutics during the mid-

---

[11]Fife, "Pioneer Mormon Remedies," p. 153. Also see Young, *The Toadstool Millionaires*, for a history of patent medicine.

[12]Dammann, *Pictorial Encyclopedia of Civil War Medical Instruments and Equipment*, *Volume II*, p. 64.

nineteenth century. Doctors prescribed stimulants or purges in the spring and fall to help the body adjust to the season. Regular physicians used diuretics, cathartics, diaphoretics and emetics as they had for centuries. They used drugs to regulate the body's internal equilibrium and to purge the system. Even so, therapeutics in the last half of the nineteenth century was changing. Poultices and mustard plasters replaced the ancient practice of counter-irritation. Bloodletting became less common.

Similarly, the pernicious practice of using mercury compounds to the point of poisoning was disappearing. More reasonable and lower doses of mercury and potassium iodide, popular since 1836, were used on a regular schedule to treat syphilis. However, Kober used potassium iodide in high doses as taught by Edward L. Keyes to "successfully" treat a gumma (a syphilitic lesion) of the brain in a woman. In contrast to other forms of syphilis which yielded to small doses of potassium iodide, Keyes taught that a gumma of the brain could be cured by high doses of the drug.[13]

The various functions the army doctors performed are best described by Dr. William C. Gorgas, nineteenth-century Surgeon-General of the U.S. Army in World War I:

> The Army Medical Officer on the plains was obliged to combine the duties of surgeon, oculist, aurist, dentist, obstetrician, general practitioner, with scanty help in nursing from the enlisted men of the Hospital Corps to whom he, himself, had taught "First Aid." He was also general health officer of the garrison; was compelled to study and inspect water supply, to plant and irrigate post gardens, and sometimes to manufacture ice. In addition, he often had a large free clinic among Indian neighbors, traders, and ranch men.[14]

---

[13]Kober, *Reminiscences*, p. 268; Keyes, *The Surgical Diseases of the Genito-Urinary Organs including Syphilis*; Keyes, *Syphilis: A Treatise for Practitioners*, pp. 147-48; and Temkin, *The Double Face of Janus and Other Essays in the History of Medicine*, p. 520.

[14]Kimball, *A Soldier-Doctor of our Army: James P. Kimball, Late Colonel and Assistant Surgeon-General, U.S. Army*, introduction.

Although Gorgas described the medical officer on the plains his description was a good summary of a doctor's duties on the high Great Basin desert.

Like medical officers today, the army surgeon generated a "mountain" of paperwork while accounting for the troops' health. He requisitioned medical and hospital supplies; kept budget records monies expended; wrote prescriptions and diet orders on each patient; supervised the steward (when he had one), the cook and other hospital workers; and enforced hospital regulations to promote health and prevent contagion by ensuring adequate ventilation and scrupulous cleanliness.

Enforcing cleanliness and sanitation was probably the post surgeon's most important duty. Many of the diseases—especially gastro-intestinal disturbances such as diarrhea—were due to poor sanitation and lack of cleanliness. Yet, he could not always count on the support of the post commander to enforce his recommendations. When surgeons William Hemphil Arthur and Frank Meachem investigated the cause of the typhoid outbreak and sent sanitation reports to the commanding officer, Meachem was ordered to stop sending the reports.[15]

On another occasion, Arthur found a soldier he was treating for typhoid fever to be moribund. Treatment consisted of repeated stimulation with one ounce of brandy every two hours. Dr. Arthur gave the nurse, a private, a bottle of brandy to comply with his orders. Later, he returned to the ward to find the patient dead and nurse drunk. Disgusted, he ordered the private to the guard house only to have the commanding officer release him with the admonishment that nursing the sick is not military duty. The commander told Arthur that he could give orders if it amused him, but the soldiers didn't have to carry them out.[16]

---

[15]Ashburn, *A History of the Medical Department of the United States Army*, p. 119.
[16]Ibid., p. 120.

The post surgeon kept extensive written records recording his duties. He kept a register of patients (Form 9), a prescription book (Form 10), a meteorological record (Form 11), record of recruits examined (Form 14), and muster and pay rolls. At the end of each month the Great Basin army surgeon wrote to the Surgeon General of the California Department, "I have the honor to report that I have been on duty as post surgeon at this station during the month ending this date per order . . ."[17] However his primary duty consisted of accompanying the troops on maneuvers and attending the wounded and sick on the battlefield and in the hospital.

Realizing the extent of the non-medical duties and the necessity for help in surgery, the hospital surgeon often looked for an assistant. At the larger forts the Surgeon General's Office assigned stewards to help in the hospital, but only rarely was a steward assigned to most Great Basin posts. The importance of the event was underlined by noting his arrival and departure in the hospital ledger.

Some surgeons like Kober at Fort McDermit persuaded soldiers assigned at their station to serve as stewards or assistants. Kober met Lieutenant Albert G. Forse when he diagnosed membranous croup in Forse's cat. Kober put the cat in a boot, administered chloroform, made an incision, inserted a chicken quill and saved the cat's life. The event sparked Forse's interest in medicine and after the episode Kober used Forse as an assistant.[18] This training could lead to a career as a surgeon; Bernard Semig, an assistant surgeon at Fort Halleck and later, at Fort McDermit, started out in the military as a steward. Also Kober started out at the age of seventeen as a steward's assistant before he attended medical school.

Later a training school for stewards was established at Fort Russell, Wyoming. George Durfee Deshon who later served

---

[17] *United States Army Regulations, of 1861, Revised*, pp. 309-12.
[18] Kober, *Reminiscences*, p. 271.

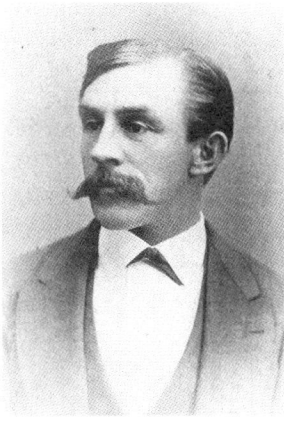

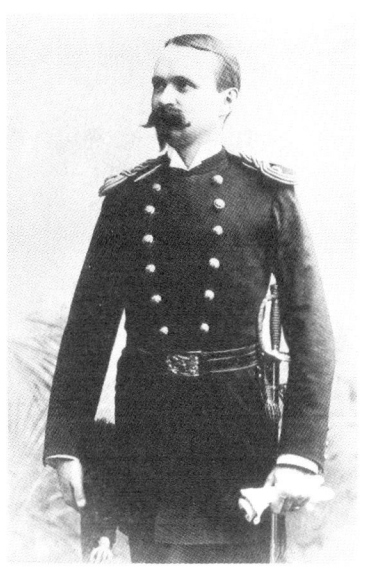

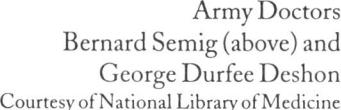

Army Doctors
Bernard Semig (above) and
George Durfee Deshon
Courtesy of National Library of Medicine

at Fort Douglas described their training when he had responsibility for the school in 1892.

> ... soldiers were instructed in anatomy, physiology, and first aid to
> prepare them for nursing in military hospitals, which were then
> wholly dependent upon enlisted men for nurses, women not being
> employed in that capacity until after the Spanish war. Soldiers
> showing adaptability were also taught Materia Medica, Pharmacy,
> Minor Surgery and Army Regulations with a view to qualifying
> them for promotion to the grade of Hospital Steward. Others were
> taught cooking. All were drilled daily in litter-bearing, ambulance
> work, tent-pitching, establishing dressing-stations, application of
> emergency bandages and tourniquets, field-cooking, and care and
> use of draft and saddle animal. The course of instruction lasted four
> months. Soldiers were admitted to the school only after having
> served a year or more in the line of the Army, to secure discipline
> and proper selection of applicants, of whom there was no dearth, as
> at that time the Hospital Corps received more pay than the Caval-

ry, Artillery, or Infantry. On completing of the course of instruc-
tion at Fort Russell the men were transferred to Post hospitals all
over the western country as vacancies occurred.[19]

When assigned to a hospital, the steward took over the
supervision of the hospital personnel such as the cook and the
matron. He also became the acting dentist and pulled teeth.[20]
A steward's duties included performing as scribe to the surgeon by taking notes on treatment, diet and admissions to the
hospital. He also filled prescription, assisted in surgery, did
dressings, and took care of emergencies and supplies.[21]

Another chore done at all hospitals entailed washing the
linen and bedding. At large forts, the surgeon general
allowed one matron per twenty patients to do the laundry,
but at smaller Great Basin posts the matron, when available,
did the laundry for the hospital and other officers besides
medical officers.[22] Sarah Winnemucca at Fort McDermit
and some enlisted men's wives at Fort Halleck performed this
function. Mrs. C. E. Oestreich in March 1876, Mrs. Frances
Kendrick in May 1876, and Mrs. Kennedy in August 1876
worked as matrons at Fort Halleck.[23]

The hospital laundresses were described in Captain
Charles King's turn-of-the-century novels as "the broods of
unkempt urchins who raced around the big black laundry
kettles that bubbled over woodfires in the backyards of Suds
Row shanties." They included "the noncommissioned officers and their red-armed wives who were the post laundresses."[24] The laundress received $2 a month for each enlisted

---

[19]Letter to Dr. J. R. Forst, February 15, 1913, from George D. Deshon. Copy supplied
by U. S. Army Medical Department Museum, Ft. Sam Houston, Texas. Also published in
Museum Notes by Army Medical Department Museum, Ft. Sam Houston.
    [20]Coffman, *The Old Army*, p. 383. The army did not provide false teeth—see Watkins
biographical sketch.
    [21]Kober, *Reminiscences*, p. 26.
    [22]*Annual Report of the Surgeon General of the Army, 1862*, p. 56.
    [23]National Archives, RG 94, E 547.
    [24]Knight, *Life and Manner in the Frontier Army*, p. 6.

men and $5 a month for officers. The position was eliminated by the Army in 1883.

At the Great Basin military hospitals there were three levels of surgeons—the civilian doctor, the commissioned officer, and during the Civil War the volunteer physician who arrived with the volunteer regiment. During the war the volunteer doctor was commissioned the same as a commissioned officer, but he was not a Regular Army officer. After the war he had three choices. He could either return to civilian practice, take the Army examination and hope to qualify as a commissioned officer or contract with the Army as a civilian physician.

The civilian doctor signed a contract for one year, but the contracts were frequently terminated by either party. Food, travel allowances and housing equivalent to a first lieutenant were allotted the contractor.

When Kober signed his first contract in 1874 he received $125 a month because duty west of the Mississippi was considered hardship and therefore paid $25 a month more than service in the East. Throughout the period of 1860-1890 the pay remained at $125 although some doctors who lived on the West Coast signed contracts for $100 a month.[25] This salary was better than that for many doctors in the United States. For instance, in New York City during the 1860s a starting doctor made $400 a year while in Massachusetts in 1850 an average salary for a doctor was $600. In contrast, more established doctors in New York City made $1,500-2,000 a year and busy police surgeons received $2,250.[26]

In the isolated West, citizens offered doctors better pay than they received in the East. For certain, contracts with guaranteed pay were an important incentive to get physicians

---

[25]National Archives, RG 94, E 561.

[26]See Starr, *The Social Transformation of American Medicine*, pp. 61-64 and p. 84; Duffy, *The Healers: The Rise of the Medical Establishment*, pp. 297-98; Rosen, *The Structure of American Medical Practice*, pp. 5-6; and Rosenberg, *Explaining Epidemics*, p 131.

to settle in their community. After Dr. John C. Handy left Camp McGarry he was guaranteed $100 per family per year by 25 families to settle in Tucson, Arizona Territory.

Other incentives were the contracts signed by the various counties to assure medical care for the indigents. Thus, in Elko, Nevada, in 1869 Dr. John Jerrold Meigs, a Harvard University graduate, in addition to pay from his regular patients received a contract for $150 per month from the county to care for patients in the "pest house."[27] In addition, the Indian Bureau gave contracts to various doctors, including military surgeons, to care for Indians living near or on military posts.

For comparison to military surgeons' pay, the U.S. Army in 1864 paid a first lieutenant $116.67 per month while privates received $13, first sergeants $22 and hospital stewards and sergeants first class got $45.[28] At the same time, civilian laborers in Texas made $1.50 a day, while in the "boom" areas of the West workers made $3 a day and up.[29] In Nevada cowboys received $25 a month.[30]

The army pay to most enlisted men was just enough to meet living expenses. As recalled by Fanny Corbusier, when the pay master arrived at Fort McDermit it was a big occasion because it happened only once a month. Sometimes, it was every two months creating hardship and debt.[31] Emphasizing its importance, the name of the paymaster and date he arrived was recorded in the hospital ledger.

Fanny, formerly a school teacher, assisted her husband in the Fort McDermit hospital and recorded this and other information in the hospital ledger.[32] The enlisted man was not the only one to feel the effects of economic hardship at the frontier

---

[27]Patterson, *Sagebrush Doctors and Health Conditions of Northeast Nevada*, p. 62.
[28]Coffman, *The Old Army*, p. 347.   [29]Ibid., p. 348.
[30]Menzies, "Where the Steer and the Antelope Play," pp. 32-33.
[31]Ibid., p. 350.   [32]Corbusier, *Verde to San Carlos*, p. 99.

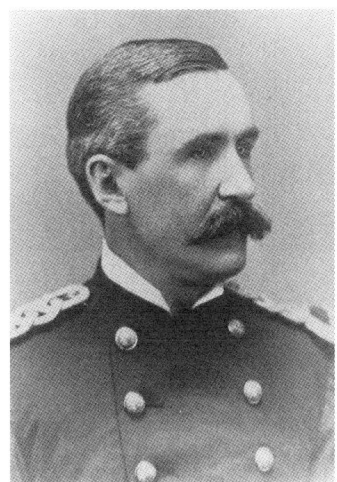

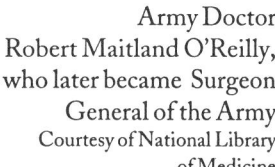

Army Doctor
Robert Maitland O'Reilly,
who later became Surgeon
General of the Army
Courtesy of National Library
of Medicine

fort. Julia Gillis, the wife of an officer at Fort Warner in 1867, recorded the situation in letters to her family:

> The merest necessaries of life cost almost fabulous prices, and although we all live in log cabins of only two rooms and have to support a style of life somewhat inferior to a washwoman or wood-sawyer, there is no one at the Post (not even the Genl) who can do more than make two ends meet.[33]

Besides pay, rank was also important—contract surgeons did not hold rank and sometimes were referred to in a derogatory manner by commissioned officers. Also commissioned medical officers advanced in rank like all other officers. Advance in rank resulted in an increase in pay while a contract surgeon's pay was virtually frozen. After receiving a commission the medical officer became an assistant surgeon (first lieutenant and captain), then, when approved by the review board and after passing the examination, became a surgeon (major) with advancement in pay.

---

[33]Gillis, *So Far from Home,* p. 158.

In 1881, Corbusier received $183.33 a month when pro-moted to captain. Those who showed promise could become a deputy surgeon general (lieutenant-colonel), and after a number of years, assistant surgeon-general (colonel).[34] A few physicians such as John Jefferson Milhau, William Hemple Arthur, Charles Smart and Robert Maitland O'Reilly became generals in the medical corps. O'Reilly became the top doctor in the army—Surgeon General of the Army.

Just as important were the retirement benefits received by regular army officers. Contract doctors were not eligible for pensions and they had to provide for their retirement by sav-ing money out of their take-home pay. Furthermore, the contract pay was only slowly increased. By the end of the cen-tury the pay for a contract doctor had increased from $100/$125 to $150 a month. However, on the whole, mili-tary doctors—both civilian and commissioned officers—received good compensation and an opportunity for income from private practice in the surrounding community. As noted, some held contracts with county hospitals in adjacent communities and others obtained contracts from the Indian Bureau.

[34]Hume, *Ornithologists of the United States Army Medical Corps*, p. 8.

Evaluation of Physicians by the Army during the Late-Nineteenth Century

Given the situation in the mid-nineteenth century (1830-1850) where anyone could hang out a sign and call himself a doctor, the Army had a difficult time obtaining competent surgeons to perform those functions required of a medical officer. The situation was aggravated when the demand increased as a result of the Civil War and the growth of hostilities in the American West. However, as early as 1848 the Army Examining Board in New York did not pass enough candidates to fill ten positions. Later in 1848 only seven of twenty-one doctors in Philadelphia passed.[1]

There were many reasons that the failure rate was so high. Some failed because of physical disabilities. Others failed because they were not citizens. Most importantly, the high failure rate was due to poor and inadequate education. Moreover, the examination was difficult and extremely stressful. This was true all the way back to the Revolutionary War when Dr. James Thacher appeared before an Army medical board in 1775. Of sixteen candidates he was one of ten who passed. He commented that the examination was "close and severe." He recalled a candidate who was asked how he would evoke a sweat in the treatment of rheumatism. The reply was, "I would have him examined by a medical committee."[2] In 1867, Dr. James Kimball took the examination and wrote:

---

[1] Brown, *The Medical Department of the United States Army from 1775 to 1873*, pp. 198-99.
[2] Thacher, *A Military Journal: 1775-1783*, p. 31.

The examination lasted a week; there were six candidates and I was the only one that passed! You can imagine it was something of an examination, as we were examined in Latin, Greek, French, and German: Arithmetic, Algebra, Geometry, Trigonometry, and Calculus, Geography, political and physical, Ancient and Modern history and Literature, Mineralogy, Conchology, Botany, and Natural Physics, etc., and then a most exhaustive examination in Medicine and all its branches.[3]

In 1885, one Harvard graduate told his teacher the examination was as hard as his initial professional exam. George Arenfed Benjamin who served at Fort Bidwell took the examination, but withdrew from further examination before the board because, "I don't feel prepared to stand a rigid examination at present."[4] Since a commission in the army was a commitment for a professional career and dismissal was difficult, the examiners had to be sure of an individual's moral character, knowledge and ability.

At the start of 1861 there were but sixty-four surgeons or assistant surgeons, including the Surgeon General and Assistant Surgeon General, in the Union Army.[5] As the Civil War progressed, causalities from battle and disease increased, resulting in an acute shortage of physicians. In 1862 Secretary of War Edwin M. Stanton informed the board that more doctors had to be commissioned. The board complied and the war effort did not suffer due to insufficient numbers of doctors.[6] At the conclusion of the war the demand subsided and the number of 1,997 acting assistant surgeons had to be drastically reduced. One year later there were only 264 doctors in the Medical Department.[7]

The recruitment of contract doctors became necessary in

[3]Kimball, *A Soldier-Doctor of Our Army*, p. 7-8.

[4]Record Group 94, Entry 561, George Benjamin.

[5]Brown, The *Medical Department of the United States Army from 1775 to 1873*, p. 215.

[6]George Worthington Adams, *Doctors in Blue: The Medical History of the Union Army in the Civil War*, p. 42.

[7]*Annual Report of the Surgeon General of the Army, 1866*, p. 383.

the late 1860s because Congress, as a result of demobilization and in an attempt to control expenses, prohibited the commissioning of medical officers. This policy also prevented candidates who had passed the examination from obtaining a commission in the medical corps. A qualified doctor wishing to make a career in the Army could only serve as a civilian contract doctor. As a result of the Congress' prohibition, the number of acting assistant surgeons or contract physicians equaled the number of assistant surgeons in the early 1870s.[8]

In order to commission more medical officers the Surgeon General reconvened examining boards to examine candidates, but the results were poor.

The tradition of a rigorous exam to keep the level of army doctors high began during the Revolutionary War, when the first military medical examining board was created. In 1875, 41 of 126 candidates passed the army examination and became commissioned officers. In 1883, 13 of 37 passed; and in 1886, 48 of 160 passed the examination given by three or four upper grade surgeons.[9] Several surgeons who served in the Great Basin were examiners on the board.

George Martin Kober, who wished to become a career army surgeon, failed the army examination in 1874, the year after he graduated from Georgetown Medical College.[10] After his military career as a contract surgeon, Kober returned to Georgetown and became a leader in hygiene and medical education. He was dean of the school from 1901-1928 and instrumental in shaping it into a leading medical college. Another easterner, Abel F. Mechem, who served at Fort Churchill, was a graduate of the University of Maryland Medical College, took the exam in 1867. He failed, and was

---

[8]Corbusier, *Verde to San Carlos:*, p. 1.

[9]Coffman, *The Old Army*, pp. 324-5 and 243.

[10]Kober Manuscript. The fact that Kober took the examination is deduced from a letter from a friend in this file asking if he had given up the idea of appearing again before the board for examination.

advised to take it again in six months, at which time he passed.[11]

Even when a doctor failed the examination, he could continue serving in a frontier military hospital as a contract doctor. Many served their entire careers in this capacity. James Ord practiced in the Army for forty-five years and Henry Haskins was a contract doctor for thirty years. His deformed leg prevented him from receiving a commission. Initially his ability to perform medical duties was questioned, but his superiors relented after he proved he could function as a surgeon.

There were others who had disabilities and served in the Army Medical Department. Several served after they had battle injuries resulting in amputations. For example, while on a scouting party against hostile Apaches in the Southwest acting Assistant Surgeon Alonzo F. Steigers was wounded in the arm requiring an amputation above the elbow. As a result the army declared him disabled, but the Secretary of War intervened and he served for twenty-one more years including sixteen months at Fort McDermit.[12] Semig was stationed at Fort McDermit and Camp Halleck after his foot was amputated as the result of an injury sustained during the Modoc War in northeastern California.

The Medical Department was sometimes so desperate to commission qualified men, that the rules were bent. Although regulations stipulated that candidates be between twenty-one and twenty-eight years of age, this requirement was waived for thirty-six-year-old Charles Knickerbocker Winne, a graduate of Jefferson Medical College, when he took the test.[13] He passed the test in 1874 and served twenty-eight years in the army.

---

[11]National Archives, RG 94, E 561

[12]Ibid., and *The Weekly Arizona Miner*, 14 January 1871, p. 3.

[13]National Archives, RG 94, E 561.

Why was it important to take the examination and have "acting" removed from the title? Once a doctor received a commission he was an officer for life and officers were seldom relieved of duty. Certainly, if he was found guilty in a court martial he could lose his commission, but the army supported its officers and few came to that end. An example of how the army supported its officers is demonstrated by Adrian Polhemus, who passed the examination between his assignments at Forts Scott and McDermit. He remained in the army until 1904, but in 1895 his commanding officer requested that he receive a four to six months leave because he was a "Confirmed victim of the cocaine and morphine habits. . . . There can be no doubt that Capt. Polhemus' usefulness as a medical officer is lost for the present, and that he is now a source of danger both directly and indirectly, and cannot be trusted."[14]

By looking at some of the examinations and reading comments about them one can get an idea about the candidate's educational background and knowledge of medicine in the late nineteenth century. First, an individual was invited to take the exam, but this usually came after he requested permission. Next, three letters of recommendation went to the board. These included statements from acquaintances about the candidate's education, training and, moral character.[15] An acquaintance, in one instance, simply stated that the candidate graduated from "Yale with honors" and included no documentation. The last step, the test, usually lasted three days and was preceded by a rigorous physical examination.

About the examination, William Hemple Arthur recalled, "The worse part of it was the very long oral examination on

---

[14]Ibid.

[15]Letters from universities were not required since only one is found in the medical personnel files in the National Archives of the 165 examined by the author and it was not from a medical school, but from an undergraduate college.

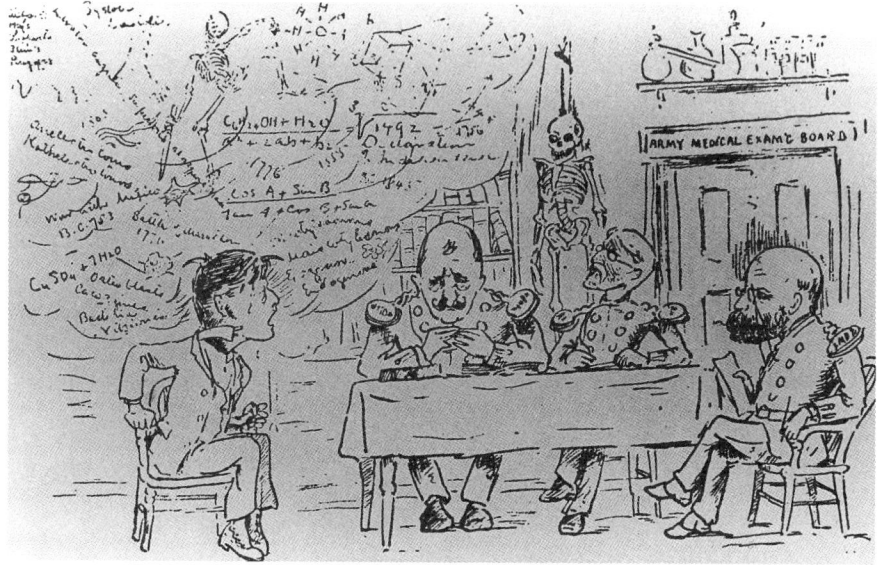

William Hemple Arthur's cartoon of the oral examination process.

Saturday for it covered not only medicine and surgery, but a large number of outside subjects as tests of general education—languages, history, geography, mathematics, literature, geology, botany, and many other subjects."[16] In other words, did the candidate have a liberal education and general knowledge in addition to an appropriate knowledge of medicine? Many of the Great Basin military surgeons had not attended college before medical school and some of those who did were poorly educated.

William Sands Newlands and Conant Bowdoin Brierly took the examination. Brierly, who served at several Great Basin forts, requested to appear before the board. A letter of recommendation in his file from H. H. Toland states Brierly

---

[16]Hume, "Admission to the Medical Department of the Army Half a Century Ago: The Experience of Brigadier-General William Hemple Arthur," p. 199.

graduated from Toland Medical College in San Francisco. The letter from the examining board in 1874 after the examination states: "Having so utterly failed in his examination before the medical examination board in this city [San Francisco] I do not consider him a capable or efficient medical officer, or a proper person to receive another contract from the Medical Department."[17] Brierly was terminated and his contract annulled. Their questions and answers demonstrate the severity of the test and how the Army dealt with the results.

Brierly did not know that Alexander the Great founded the Macedonian Empire; that, according to legend, Romulus and Remus founded the Roman Empire; that Charlemagne was King of the Franks and the first Germanic ruler of the Romans; and the Vikings, Normans and Henry VIII of England conquered Ireland; and that the Romans conquered Wales. He did not know that an artesian well is a well in which the water rises above the level of the water in the ground, or that it takes the moon 29½ days to make one revolution around the earth. He also did not know who discovered America.

On the other hand, Newlands did know the heliocentric and geocentric theories of light and correctly named the divisions of the animal kingdom.[18] In addition, he knew that diatones and infusoria are lower forms of the protozoa; that whales, porpoises and walruses are examples of marine mammals, that the subdivisions of the vertebrates included birds . . . ; and that the succession of the seasons is explained by the obliquity of the earth to the ecliptic path of the sun in the heavens. He was able to give the parts of speech; correctly define a fraction; and recall the principle rivers in the United States.[19]

---

[17]Ibid.

[18]The heliocentric theory placed the sun at the center of the universe while the geocentric theory considered the earth to be the center of the universe.

[19]National Archives, RG 94, E 561.

These questions would seem fair and good indicators of a candidate's general knowledge. An educated and informed nineteenth-century person was expected to know the answers. Nonetheless, medical knowledge was more important to the soldier living in isolation on the vast deserts of the Great Basin. The following are examples of medical-related questions that Brierly failed to answer or at all:

• How are the short bones divided? *Answer:* "I don't know."
• What muscles are attached to the coccyx? *Answer:* "I don't know."
• What muscles are attached to lesser trochanter? *Answer:* "I don't know."
• Pathology: *Examiner's comment:* "Knew nothing of pathology."
• Practice of Medicine: [Knew of digitalis but thought it was a sedative used for Rheumatism and fevers.] *Examiner's comment:* "Of disease of heart and lungs he knew nothing."
• Obstetrics: *Examiner's comment:* "Gave a very general and vague description of the mechanism of labor, with many inaccuracies."
• Toxicology: *Examiner's comment:* "Very limited knowledge of subject."
• What is the composition of blood? *Answer:* "I cannot give it."[20]

In contrast, Edward Corson's medical examination consists of twenty-six pages of written answers showing a high degree of medical knowledge, but unfortunately, he was eliminated due to his past history of alcoholism.[21] Excerpts from his medical examination include an accurate description of: the radius [a bone in the forearm]; the posterior tibial artery [an artery in the leg] and its distribution; and the ligaments of the hip joint, pointing out the relative importance of each. Other medical-related questions included questions on:

• Physiology: He accurately described digestion and the value of the different kinds of food; the circulation of the blood; the nutrition of the fluids and solids of the body; and the function of the blood and its vitality.
• Hygiene: 1. How can a soldier best preserve his health? *Answer:* "[By]

[20]Ibid.   [21]Ibid.

regulation of the quality, quantity, and character of his food and drink: attention to the kind and amount of clothing, the location of his camp and post as regards climatic influences; the amount of exercise and duty, mental divisions of general morale bathing and cleanliness to avoid overcrowding and the generation of occlusive exposure after night, and to the influence of malaria. The food should be frequently varied and consist of nitrogenous, nonnitrogenous and inorganic proximate principles, both animal and vegetable, with a sufficient amount of fresh vegetables and the vegetable acids, The accessory principles of food as coffee, tobacco, tea, alcohol et cet. should be furnished at proper times and in proper quantities. They will take the place of food when the latter is unobtainable, and prevent as dangerous a rapid waste of tissues during forced marches, . . . Water containing a large amount of earthy matters will produce diarrhoea at first as the water of our large rivers of the west, but this will last but for a short time. Water containing a minute quantity of lead is highly poisonous; rain-water and soft water dissolve lead, but the addition of a minute quantity of a sulphate will prevent this, and render water passing over lead harmless . . . Water may be purified by boiling, distilling, filtration through charcoal, sand or gravel, or by the permanganate of potash, quick-lime, alum albumien. Water should never be drank very cold after the system has commenced to cool following over-heating . . . Troops should never have fatiguing work before breakfast or at least their coffee, or should they be drilled under a very hot sun . . . the soldier should bathe twice daily, and the shower-bath is highly beneficial."

• Hygiene: 2. What impurities are found in the air? *Answer:* ". . . Sulpuretted hydrogen, in the vicinities of privies, latrines, decaying vegetable matters, and sewers, it may be detected by a soluble salt of lead. carbonic acid found in the bottom of wells, . . . Carburetted hydrogen is exhaled from marshes and may escape from the light supply of buildings or street tubes. Ozone, a hygienic agent capable of destroying organic matters and produced by electricity. It is a powerful antiseptic. . . . "

• Hygiene: 3. What are the most important antiscorbutics? *Answer:* ". . . The diet to prevent scurvy should be changed that it may not become monotonous and should contain fresh vegetables, especially the onion, potatoe [*sic*], turnip and carrot. None of the laws of hygiene should be broken . . . lemon and lime juice."

The hygiene of soldiers was a very important part of the

frontier surgeon's responsibilities and Corson's answers give insight into his thoughts about the use of tobacco, coffee, tea and alcohol. His concept of "earthy matters" in water causing diarrhea reflects nineteenth-century theory of disease and he understood the necessity of purification. He also pointed out that lead poisoning resulted from drinking rain water that leached lead out of roof gutters and pipes. Equally or more important for the frontier soldier, he knew how to prevent scurvy.

Practice of Medicine questions included:

1. What is scorbutus [scurvy], its course, cause, symptoms and treatment? Answer: "It is primarily a blood-disease, as consisting in a deficiency in some of the constituents of the blood, especially of the salts of potash, and in a deterioration of the others as albumien and fibrin; and secondarily a disease of the tissues from a deficiency in their nutritive supply. Its first symptom is great fatigue following ordinary labor, which change in temper and character of the individual; he becomes very irritable and shows a disinclination for duty and ordinary pursuits. The tissues bleed freely from slight wounds and cicatricial tissue ulcerates. The gums becomes soft, springy, and bleeding; the teeth loosen in their sockets and fall out; the hair falls out and the skin is rough and leparous. Purpura or hemorrhagic spots appear over the body; the breath is foul and faetid. The causes of Scorbutus are, a sameness of diet, combined with unhygienic surroundings; exposure to cold, dampness, darkness, mental depression following loss, defeat of battle, bad news et cet; homesickness and especially the absence of fresh vegetables."

2. Write a prescription suitable for chronic or habitual constipation.

    Write a prescription for general tonic purposes where anaemia exists.

    Write one to promote diaphoresis.

    Write one to promote diuresis.

These prescriptions reflect common conditions and treatment of that time (1874). It was still acceptable to treat disease by purging the system by diaphoresis (sweating) and diuresis (increased urine production). Corson answered these questions correctly.

Surgery questions included:

1. Describe simple ulcer of the lip, with treatment. *Answer:* "Simple ulcer of the lip if very persistent, becomes painful, very annoying, and depends upon a low state of the system. It will generally yield to tonics, exercise, and the local application of the nitrate of silver."
2. Describe a gunshot wound of the arm, implicating the upper third and head of the humerus; but not wounding the main blood vessels of the part; with treatment and prognosis as well as operation needed, and describe the manner of performing it. *Answer:* ". . . involving the shoulder joint, and might be complicated with a dislocation of the head of the humerus. This wound would be best treated by resection of the head of the humerus, and the prognosis would be that the patient would recover with quite a useful limb with all necessary motion. The operation should be performed as follows: after the administration of anesthetic, the bullet wound should be enlarged over the head of the bone, all foreign matters removed and the head and neck of the humerus resected, the extent being according to the extent of the injury."[22]

The ulcer discussed by Corson is now known to be due to the herpes simplex virus, and he knew the symptoms and treatment. The treatment he prescribed was used until twenty or thirty years ago. His answer to the treatment for a gun shot wound to the arm reflects his technical knowledge. Twenty years earlier and without the use of anesthesia the answer might have simply been amputation.

[22]Ibid.

Diseases of Soldiers
Stationed in the Great Basin

Introduction

During the early years of military presence in the Intermountain West, 1861-1865—the Civil War years—service-
men in the East had a higher mortality and morbidity rate
from disease than soldiers and male civilians in the West.[1]
The health conditions in the East reflected inadequate sanitation and poor hygiene due to crowding and conditions during war. In the West, living conditions were more healthful
due to less contamination of the environment and the good
climate.

Later, military surgeons commented on the salubrious
effect of the climate and altitude on the health of the command. For instance, Surgeon Edward P. Vollum at Fort Douglas in 1874 noted that he and the local physicians observed
the beneficial effect of Utah's climate on phthisis (tuberculosis) and asthma. In a report to the Surgeon General he stated
that there were no cases of phthisis that are "unconnected
with heredity transmission." Furthermore, early cases of
tuberculosis "get well spontaneously from the beneficial
effects of the altitude and the inland dry character of the
atmosphere." He continued: "The beneficial influence of this
climate on asthma is decided, and deserves a prominent
mention."[2] These observations re-enforced Henry I.

---

[1] Shryock, "A Medical Perspective on the Civil War," pp. 164.

[2] *Circular No. 8*, p. 340-343.

Bowditch's 1862 observations that pulmonary phthisis was more frequent in low damp localities than on higher land.[3]

On the other side of the Great Basin similar comments were made. In June 1867 at Fort Independence, Matthews stated that there was "One trifling case on sick-report during the month."[4] In 1873 at Fort Warner, there were three to six on sick report a month and an average strength of fifty men.[5] In all, most soldiers enjoyed good health at the Great Basin commands.

Sanitation, hygiene and adequate food supplies were still a problem for the soldiers stationed there. Doctors did not understand the role of the mosquito in malaria and the role of fomites in the spread of some disease had not been elucidated.[6] As a result, food, water and utensils were sometimes contaminated; bad habits extended and increased the risk. In this environment epidemics of dysentery or diarrhea such as cholera, typhoid and other enteric diseases were a threat to military camps and the civilian population.

Other diseases such as rheumatic fever spread in epidemic proportions through the West partly because the importance of the "contagious" sore throat was not associated with the severe arthritis. Frequent questions on the military examination for doctors emphasized concern about these issues. Thus, poor hygiene, uncleanliness and spread of contaminated material were the most important factors in the spread of infectious diarrhea, the most prevalent disorder on the western frontier.

After diarrhea and other epidemic diseases the surgeon spent most of his time treating more mundane problems. By reviewing the hospital records one can get an idea of the day-to-day practice at Forts Churchill, Bidwell, Halleck, Inde-

---

[3]Medical Committee of the Massachusetts Medical Society, v. X, No. 11, 1862.

[4]National Archives, RG 94, E 547, B 135, p. 267.

[5]Ibid., B. 327-328.

[6]Fomites are physical objects that carry bacteria resulting in the spread of disease.

pendence, McDermit and other Great Basin posts.[7] During 1860 and 1861 the aggregate strength of Fort Churchill varied from 182 to 284 while admissions to the hospital varied from 23 to 70 per month. During one month an outbreak of diarrhea and other diseases hospitalized 34 percent of the command with an average length of stay of three days leaving no doubt that the hospital was full and the strength of the command was, on occasion, depleted.

Between 1870 and 1874 health conditions at seven Great Basin forts—Cameron, Bidwell, Douglas, Halleck, Harney, Independence and McDermit—were reported to the Surgeon General. At Fort Cameron, the mean strength of the command varied between 181 and 215 men and upper respiratory infections led the list with 11 cases.

Although respiratory infections were, from time to time, a problem in the Great Basin, diarrhea was a greater threat to life. Fort Douglas had an average of 364 men and diarrhea was the most common disease with 836 cases over a four year period. Trauma from accidents with 671 cases, malarial fever with 472 and rheumatism with 400 were next in frequency.

Later in the 1890s when six hundred were stationed at Fort Douglas, Assistant Surgeon Deshon reported "The hospital averaged about twenty patients, the commonest causes of admission being tonsillitis, rheumatic affections, venereal [disease] and trauma. On the other hand, obstetric and children's disease constituted the bulk of the work among the civilians for the Army doctor."[8]

At Fort Halleck with a mean strength of 99 men and four to six officers, the most common cause for sick call was trauma (152 cases during the same period). Harney had mean strength of 56 and trauma was also the most common disor-

---

[7]National Archives, RG 94, E 574. Also see *Circular No. 8*, p. 511.

[8]Letter to Dr. J. R. Forst, February 15, 1913, from George D. Deshon. Copy supplied by U. S. Army Medical Department Museum, Ft. Sam Houston, Texas. Also published in Museum Notes by Army Medical Department Museum, Ft. Sam Houston.

der with 176 cases. Fort Independence had a mean strength of 48-63, and rheumatism and accidents were equal with 40 cases each. For the same period at McDermit the mean strength was 59 men with two to three officers, fever led the list with 103 cases. Thus, each fort had unique problems, but none was immune to alcoholism, intestinal disorders and other disease that from time to time occurred.

To keep uniform statistics and to simplify reporting of the various illnesses, the Surgeon General's Office classified diseases in four categories: General Disease A (typho-malarial fever, remittent fever, intermittent fever and other diseases of this group), General Disease B (rheumatism, syphilis, consumption, and other diseases of this group), Local Diseases (catarrh and bronchitis, pneumonia, pleurisy, diarrhea, hernia, gonorrhea, alcoholism and other diseases of this group) and Violent Diseases and Deaths. General Disease A and B were infectious diseases readily identified in all army installations. Local Diseases with the exception of alcoholism, gonorrhea, and hernia appear to be local outbreaks of acute infectious disease as a result of close living conditions in barracks. Violent Diseases, on the other hand, reflect the prevalence of accidents associated with soldiering and life on the frontier.

Over the four year period there were 1,477 men per year on sick call (not including trauma) at the seven bases (Cameron, Bidwell, Douglas, Halleck, Harney, Independence and McDermit). The average number of men stationed at these combined bases was approximately 969 producing a sick rate of 1,524 per 1,000 men. During this period the sick rate for the whole United States Army varied from a high of 2,087 in 1871 to a low of 1,561 in 1873.[9] Therefore, the military sick rate on the Great Basin appeared to be at the low end of the average for the Army.

---

[9]Ashburn, *A History of the Medical Department of the United States Army*, p.113.

A further breakdown of the specific illnesses during this early period reveals diarrhea with 1,271 entries in the hospital records of the seven forts, accounting for 18.4 percent of the cases. Trauma accounted for 1,257 (18.2%) of the cases; malarial fevers were 835 (12.1%) and rheumatism resulted in 658 (9.5%) entries. Although alcoholism accounted for an epidemic high percentage of the admissions, overall it was 3.6 percent. Another social problem among soldiers, venereal disease, was less than one half as prevalent as alcoholism. In an interesting observation, Kober in unpublished memoirs figured that as high as 15 percent of the soldiers who reported for sick call would not have complained of their illness in civilian life.[10]

A word of caution is necessary about prevalence of disease in the nineteenth century because some diseases were confused with each other. The diarrhea seen with scurvy was confused with the diarrhea of gastro-intestinal disease while scurvy-associated arthritis was confused with other causes of joint pain and stiffness of the lower extremities. Also, fever and malaise associated with many infectious diseases sometimes overshadowed the more diagnostic features resulting in misdiagnosis.

Thus, malaria in camps during the Spanish-American War of 1898 was often confused with typhoid fever. In Baltimore during the Great Basin frontier era, there was lack of uniformity in diagnosis of these two disorders. For instance in 1897, the ratio of death rates for typhoid and malaria was 1:16 at Johns Hopkins Hospital while in the city the ratio was 1:1. Obviously, the discrepancies were due to other factors than patient selection. The differences in criteria for diagnosis were significant.[11] Even so, the Surgeon General's classification emphasized the important causes for morbidity

[10]Kober Manuscript, p. 125.

[11]Ackerknecht, *Malaria in the Upper Mississippi Valley 1760-1900*, p. 7.

in the Great Basin commands. The following paragraphs give a historical perspective of the most common illnesses in Great Basin forts.

INTERMITTENT AND OTHER MALARIAL FEVERS

The malaria parasite caused intermittent fever that was widespread across nineteenth-century America and Nevada. In fact, malaria was transmitted by the Anopheles mosquito in all areas of the country except the far north, the high mountains and the deserts of the West. Even though *Anopheles freeborni*, a vector for malaria, was present in parts of Nevada and the Great Basin during the nineteenth century, the conditions necessary for its survival and propagation were not common.[12] The female Anopheles mosquito that harbored the parasite thrived in areas where there was stagnate and swampy water, a condition prevalent along the rivers and streams in the Central Valley of California, but rare in Nevada.

Dr. James L. Tyson in 1849 described the swarms of mosquitoes in the Sacramento Delta which almost drove his party "mad." He observed, "most of us presented the appearance of a recent recovery from small-pox." As a consequence, he suffered from a "raging fever" that yielded to treatment by "Dr. P. of Baltimore."[13]

Fortunately, for the new inhabitants of the Great Basin, the dry, hot seasons restricted the distribution of the mosquito.[14] Therefore, most of the afflicted individuals in the Great Basin came from endemic areas in the Midwest, East, South, and California. Surgeon Richard A. Powell at Fort Warner

---

[12]The information regarding the presence of *Anopheles freeborni* in Nevada was obtained from the state entomologist at the Nevada Department of Agriculture. According to Russell, *Man's Mastery of Malaria*, p. 175-76, *A. freeborni* was the vector of "miner's fever" during the gold rush days in California.

[13]Tyson, *Diary of a Physician in California*, pp. 67 and 100.

recognized that all of the soldiers who came down with malarial fevers had been stationed in Virginia and did not contact the illness in the Great Basin. During his tenure at the fort the disease was devastating: "About three-fourths of the garrison have been sick [November 1867] with Remittent and Intermittent fevers. . . , Dr. Powell has applied for change of station for himself; he says we are so high in the mountains here, he will never get well."[15]

The surgeon at Fort Douglas in 1869 recognized that the members of the 7th Infantry with malaria had contracted the disease in Florida.[16] However, the malaria parasite dates to the time of Columbus.

Before Columbus and his men stepped ashore and introduced malaria to America, the Indians were free of the disease.[17] One half of the new colony of Jamestown died of ague—the English term for malaria. By the mid-17th century malaria was well entrenched in the American colonies. Slowly and steadily it was carried into the Mississippi Valley and beyond.[18] The killer parasites—*Plasmodium vivax* and *P. falciparum*—swept the country with devastating results.[19] Thousands died in the Ohio and Mississippi river valleys; and in the Northwest 90 percent of the Columbia River Valley Native Americans died in 1828 during an epidemic.[20]

Characteristically, malaria began in childhood. Depending on the type of parasite, the child's resistance and degree of infection, a debilitating and anemic condition that can last a life time might develop. The benign form, vivax malaria,

---

[14]To this day, the mosquitoes in parts of the Great Basin (for instance, Warner Valley) remain horrible, in vast number, and, vicious!

[15]Gilliss, *So Far From Home*, p. 158.

[16]"Fort Douglas Medical History," Fort Douglas Museum, Salt Lake City.

[17]Warshaw, *Malaria: The Biography of a Killer*, p. 25.

[18]Duffy, *Epidemics in Colonial America*, pp. 205-206.

[19]The English introduced Plasmodium vivax and P. malariae into the American continent at Jamestown in 1607 while slaves from Africa brought P. falciparum to the colonies in 1620. Oakes, Jr., *Malaria: Obstacles and Opportunities*, p. 38.

[20]Ibid., pp. 26-30.

recurs every other day in a cycle known as tertian. In contrast, falciparum—malignant tertian—could cause "brain fever" and death. In actuality, most cases were not characteristic in their fever cycle and were mixed infections. These infections characterized by intermittent fever produced an enlarged spleen, yellowish skin and a periodic fever. Some patients suffered recurrent paroxysms of fever and chills every four days, hence the designation, quotidian fever. Depending on the malarial parasite the "shaking chill" and fever recurred one to four days.

When properly diagnosed the treatment of malaria in the late-nineteenth century was one of relative success. Since 1633 when cinchona bark was introduced in Europe, various forms of quinine were used successfully to treat malarial fevers.[21] Unfortunately, the cinchona tree grew only in remote South America making the treatment expensive. Not until the nineteenth century was the active ingredient, quinine, isolated from the bark by Pierre Joseph Pelletier and Joseph Bienaime Caventou.

In 1838 Surgeon Benjamin Franklin Harney, the medical director of the Army in Florida started the use of "sulphate of quina" in large doses for the treatment of intermittent fever. The Civil War removed any doubts concerning the effectiveness of quinine.[22] As a result of this knowledge of quinine, Great Basin military doctors successfully treated intermittent fever.

By 1865, the mortality rate in the United States was still approximately 60 per 1,000 cases.[23] In the 1870s, malaria peaked as a cause of death.[24] By 1875, the statistics from the Great Basin forts show a significant decrease in the illness.

---

[21]Ibid., p. 178.

[22]Smith, "Quinine and Fever: The Development of the Effective Dosage," pp. 363 and 366.

[23]Faust, "Clinical and Public Health Aspects of Malaria...., p. 187.

[24]Ackerknecht, *Malaria in the Upper Mississippi Valley 1760-1900*, p. 60.

Unfortunately, the price of quinine remained high until 1880 (In 1860, it was $1.20-1.80 per ounce; 1870, $2.20-2.40; 1880, $2.20-3.20; 1890, $0.39-0.42.) when the price markedly declined.[25] In actuality, treatment with quinine did not always produce a cure by killing all of the parasites, but it did produce clinical improvement.

In spite of the fact that malaria was not transmitted in the Great Basin, it was the most prevalent disease at Fort Churchill. During the two year period, 1868-1869, at Camp Bidwell malarial fever was the most common illness causing 25 percent of the hospitalizations while at Camp Independence during the same period of time it was third (18%) behind diarrheal diseases (29%) and rheumatic fever (19%).[26]

Even though quinine cured clinical malaria, the victim of intermittent fever might be left in a debilitated and weakened condition. To further complicate the picture, doctors were not able to diagnose the disorder with complete accuracy. Hepatitis, lumbago and other febrile illnesses confused the clinical diagnosis. Typhoid fever was frequently confused with malaria and was called typho-malaria.

Another frequently diagnosed fever in the nineteenth century was mountain fever. It is difficult to determine if this was a specific illness, and more likely it was a mixed bag of diseases. In Idaho the term eventually became associated with Rocky Mountain Spotted Fever, a tick-borne rickettsial disease. Kober considered it synonymous with typho-malaria fever that readily yielded to a mild cathartic, Dover's powder, and five grain doses of quinine three or four times a day.[27] Many cases of mountain fever were typhoid fever since their occurrence usually coincided—late summer and fall.[28] On

---

[25]Ibid., p. 113.
[26]*Circular No. 4*, pp. 446 and 450. Also, note that trauma and accidents were not included in the reports from Bidwell and Independence.
[27]Kober Manuscript, pp. 117-18.
[28]Richards, *Of Medicine, Hospitals, and Doctors*, p. 21.

the other hand, mountain fever in some situations was confused with malaria.

However, the definitive diagnoses of malaria had to await until 1880 when Charles Louis Alphonse Laveran demonstrated the parasite in the blood of patients with the characteristic fever. Then, the accuracy of diagnosis increased and treatment became more successful leaving diarrheal diseases alone at the top of the pyramid as the most prevalent illness on the frontier.

DIARRHEAL DISEASES

Diarrhea and dysentery were symptoms of diseases that were common in the nineteenth-century West. It has been calculated that intestinal disease, present in soldiers and civilians alike, was the most common disorder on the frontier. In Sacramento, California, in 1850 diarrhea was known as "the disease of California."[29] California's mild climate was blamed for the most prevalent illnesses: diarrhea and intermittent fever. They were endemic in the mining camps and new communities that sprang up in northern California.[30] The condition of diarrhea was so frequent that the disorder was not considered a disease unless disability resulted.

Even so, it was second to "the fever" at Fort Churchill in 1860-1861.[31] Seventy-seven patients, or twelve percent of those admitted during the hospital's first eighteen months of operation were suffering from diarrhea. This did not include admissions for other intestinal disorders such as colica, hemorrhoids, and constipation. During epidemics of diarrhea, the disorder surpassed intermittent fever as the most common ailment.

---

[29]Read, "Diseases, Drugs and Doctors on the Oregon-California Trail in the Gold-Rush years," p. 276.

[30]Nunis, *A Medical Journey in California by Dr. Pierre Garnier*, p. 38.

[31]National Archives, RG 94, Churchill Returns. The 94 patients includes 8 cases of hepatitis.

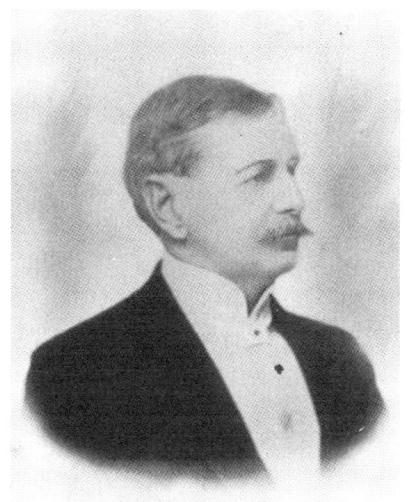

Army Doctor
Charles Carroll Furley
Courtesy of Wichita-Sedwick
County Historical Museum

Generally, most bacterial diarrhea is little more than debilitating and inconvenient. According to Dr. Charles Furley at Fort Churchill they readily yielded to treatment, but some, like typhoid and cholera, were a threat to life. Cholera frequently resulted in death from dehydration within twenty-four hours while typhoid resulted in a slower death from septicemia.[32] Cholera swept the West in 1866-1867 appearing in San Francisco and in Kansas.[33] Later, after completion of the Central Pacific Railroad in 1869, cholera appeared in Sacramento, Elko, Salt Lake City, and other communities along the line. However, during this period doctors treated only a handful of patients with acute gastroenteritis—known as cholera morbus—at military posts in the western Great Basin.[34]

[32]Septicemia is the condition when the bacteria spreads to the blood.

[33]*Circular No. 5.*, p. XIII.

[34]National Archives, RG 94, E 574. Cholera morbus was acute gastroenteritis and not the usual fatal disease now known as Asiatic cholera.

ACUTE RHEUMATISM

Next, in prevalence during the early frontier military years behind intermittent fever and diarrhea was acute rheumatism. In contrast, chronic rheumatism now known as osteoarthritis, was a disorder of old age. Today, the acute form is no longer referred to as acute rheumatism, but is recognized as rheumatic fever and is caused by the bacterium, *Group A Beta Streptococcus*.

In 1882 Dr. Morris Longstreth, lecturer in pathological anatomy at Jefferson Medical College, described acute rheumatism as "a group of symptoms . . . having a common or supposed common cause . . . without . . . any . . . anatomical basis." There were many theories as to the cause and the "recent popular" germ or infectious theory had many proponents. As evidence Longstreth pointed out that its complications included involvement of the serous membranes (pleural, pericardial and endocardial) similar to other infectious diseases, and that it occurred in epidemics following scarlet fever.[35]

Scarlet fever, the initial infection that could lead to rheumatic fever, was a serious threat in early Nevada and occurred with devastating consequences: possible death. In May 1875, the illness raged throughout Humboldt County, in July it spread to Battle Mountain, in November it was rampant in Paradise Valley, but by Christmas the epidemic had abated.[36]

Nevertheless, the initial event in acute rheumatism, the sore throat, was recognized as "rheumatic angina," but it was only one of the many symptoms associated with the disease. As would be expected, doctors frequently saw tonsillitis at

---

[35]See Longstreth, *Rheumatism, Gout, and Some Allied Disorders*, for the details.

[36]*The Silver State*, May 19, 1875, 3;3; July 3, 1875, 3;1; Nov. 3, 1875, 3;1; and Dec. 23, 1875, 3;1.

the fort hospital. Fortunately, death occurred only rarely during an acute episode of acute rheumatism. Mortality was more common from the later associated heart disease. Repeated attacks damaged the heart valves producing an enlarged heart and heart failure. Assistant Surgeon John B. Porter suffered epileptic seizures as a result of his rheumatic fever and died in 1869 at Fort Douglas from the associated heart disease.

Initially, in 1860, treatment consisted of the administration of alkaline bases such as nitrate of potash, bicarbonate of potash, or citrate of potash in a combination with mineral or carbonic acid. Most diseases at that time were treated with an average of two prescriptions. Longstreth found that bromide of potash, introduced in 1865, had "merits" and "good effects."[37] Up to the 1870s, the treatment of the pain associated with arthritis was not entirely successful. Then, a breakthrough occurred, treatment with salicyl.

Although salicin was discovered in the first third of the nineteenth century, it was too expensive to produce. The bark of the willow tree (genus *Salix*) from which it was derived was used since Antiquity for pain relief. Its relative, salicylic acid, was first used and described in Traube's Berlin Clinic in 1876.[38] Longstreth felt that salicylic acid was destructive of the rheumatism poison, but more importantly, it readily ameliorated the painful symptoms.

The toxic symptoms of salicylic acid were well known in the nineteenth century. However, acetylsalicylic acid (aspirin), a related compound, was developed in 1898 by Bayer. It is still effective in controlling the joint pain associated with acute rheumatic fever. For many years, well into the twentieth century, doctors used aspirin to a toxic level—ringing in the ears—and then, decreased the dose to a mainte-

---

[37]Longstreth, *Rheumatism, Gout, and Some Allied Disorders*, p. 204.   [38]Ibid., p. 205.

nance level in order to control the pain, fever, and inflammatory manifestations of the disease.

TRAUMA

Accidents and violence were near the top of the list of illnesses treated at the Great Basin military hospitals. Soldiers,
ranchers and miners, hardy as they were, nevertheless were
involved in activities that carried a high risk of trauma and
death. In addition they were around unpredictable and haz-
ardous horses. A runaway horse was a threat to more than
limb and bone. Skull fractures, intracerebral hemorrhage,
spinal cord injuries, and chest and abdominal trauma could
result in death. If the patient survived the accident, amputation with postoperative infection due to poor aseptic technique could result.

Fort Harney had the highest accident rate during the period from 1870 to 1874 with an average of forty-four cases per
year. The fort had a mean strength of fifty-six men. At Fort
Churchill in the early 1860s, trauma of all types, including
"accidents, a fracture or dislocation which are the certain
sequences of mounting cavalry on Spanish Stock"—accounted for 10 percent of the hospitalizations.[39]

Not to be ignored is the part guns and knives played in
trauma. Miners and cowboys as well as soldiers carried arms
and used them with the slightest provocation, often under
the influence of alcohol, to settle a dispute or argument. Private Edward Conlin was asleep in his bed when his protago-
nist murdered him at Fort Bidwell on February 24, 1874.[40]
Accidental shootings also occurred. Dr. Pierre Garnier
described the frontier fascination with guns when he wrote,
"The Yankees especially have the deplorable habit of playing

---

[39]Record Group 92, Churchill Returns.
[40]Record Group 94, Entry 547, Book 101, p. 109.
[41]Garnier, *A Medical Journey in California*, p. 60.

with their revolvers, five or six-shot repeaters, the way South Americans play with their daggers."[41] With eight year's experience in the West, including three at Fort Douglas, Assistant Surgeon William Cline Borden similarly wrote: ". . . while I saw the revolver prettly [*sic*] frequently worn for ornamental purposes, I never knew it to be used otherwise, and my only experience of bloodshed from one was when called professionally to see a cowboy, who had accidentally shot himself in the leg with his own ornament."[42]

In some communities guns were used for more than ornaments. Arguments, under the influence of alcohol, were many times settled with guns. Dr. Henry Bergstein recalled the early days of Pioche when "the crack of the revolver and knife-wounds were daily heard and seen."[43]

On the other hand, trauma—including gunshot wound—from the frontier Indian wars was a rarity in the Great Basin. During Nevada's twenty-eight-year period of military presence, the United States Army only recognized six regular army battles and these, not including the Pyramid Lake battle, were minor compared to battles in the adjacent territories of Utah, California, Oregon and Idaho. However, a surgeon was always necessary. The *Humboldt Register* describes Dr. Thomas H. Snow's performance on a battlefield in northern Nevada:

> Dr. Snow, a citizen physician accompanying the detachment from Company I, will be long remembered and loved by the gallant men who fought that day. He rode over all parts of the field during the battle, attending to the wounded soldiers where they fell, applying the antidotes necessary to destroy the deadly effect produced by poisoned arrows—which if not attended to at once must prove fatal. An old man, whose head is white with the frost of many Winters, but whose heart is as warm and his energies as vigorous as those of a youth, he braved the perils of frost and battle to alleviate

---

[42]Borden, "William Cline Borden 1858-1934," p. 2.
[43]Davis, *The History of Nevada*, p. 610.

the suffering of his fellow man. May God protect him, is the soldiers prayer.[44]

Although skirmishes with Native Americans in Nevada
were usually minor, troops from Forts Halleck and McDermit were dispatched in 1873 against the Modoc tribe led by
Captain Jack in northeastern California; to Idaho to fight
against Chief Joseph and the Nez Perce in 1877; to Oregon
in 1878 against the Bannocks; and to Arizona in 1883
against the Apaches. In these battles the doctors treated
many gun shot and arrow wounds.

SMALLPOX

Smallpox is a viral disease similar to measles in that its
most visible effect is the pronounced skin eruption. Both
were deadly on the frontier, especially among the American
Indians, but smallpox had a higher mortality in the immi-
grant community. After 1796 smallpox, endemic and frequently epidemic, was preventable by vaccination.

In the Great Basin as in other parts of the world, this was
one disease where doctors had a significant impact. The story

---

[44]*The Humboldt Register,* January 20, 1866, 2; 3. Although it appears that the story of
Snow is dramatized, much has been written about poisoned arrows. According to Bill,
"Notes on Arrow Wounds," p. 368, poisoned arrows were made by exposing the liver of an
animal to a rattlesnake bite. The animal is killed, the liver is buried in the skin for a week and
then dug up. The arrow is dipped in the putrefying mass, dried, dipped in blood and used
when dry. He describes a horse dying after being shot with a poison arrow, but has never
known a man to so die. The Indians in Nevada are described in the *Handbook of North American Indians,* v. 11, p. 79, as using similar techniques to poison arrows, but no specific
descriptions are given of the effect of poison arrows on humans. Dr. William H. Corbusier
concluded that most of the poisonous effect of arrow wounds was due to filth and delayed
care in treatment. He described the following method used by the Indians in Arizonia Territory to poison their war arrows. "The skinned and dried head of a rattlesnake was powdered on a stone and mixed with any clotted blood, salt and a liquid squeezed from large red
ants, or the ants themselves dried and powdered. This mixture was allowed to stand for a
time and then carefully smeared on the arrowheads with a piece of buckskin, and in order to
distinguish them from untreated arrows, they were dipped in a stinking liquid obtained by
crushing certain leaves." Dr. Corbusier also related that an Indian informed him that poisonous insects, including spiders, were sometimes used to make the poisonous concoction.
Corbusier, *Verde to San Carlos,* pp. 21-23.

of smallpox at Great Basin military bases was one of success. Surgeon Charles C. Furley reported that two new recruits at Fort Churchill in June 1862 developed the contagion, but vaccination of the command prevented its spread. In February and March 1863 he vaccinated 550 Native Indians against smallpox and treated 230 for various skin diseases, bronchitis and fevers at the post.[45]

Smallpox's presence in communities near military bases caused concern, and alarmed the military surgeon to the possibility of spread to the base. In September 1867, Virginia City recorded three or four cases and one death.[46] Again in 1869 and 1881 cases appeared on the Comstock.[47] Doctors in Austin, Nevada, treated several cases in 1869, but Austin and Virginia City were far removed from the military bases.[48] However, when the disease appeared in Elko in January 1869 with a mortality of three to five a day, the doctor at Fort Halleck became alarmed and vaccinated all of the soldiers at the base. Consequently, no cases appeared at Fort Halleck.[49] At the same time smallpox was a concern in Salt Lake City; 221 men of the 36th Infantry were vaccinated.[50] In the spring of 1874, smallpox again appeared in Elko. At Fort Halleck a soldier who probably was inadequately immunized had a mild case.[51] When smallpox appeared in Silver City, Idaho, the surgeon vaccinated sixty-six soldiers at Fort McDermit.[52]

Vaccination was accomplished by obtaining varicella (cowpox) material dried on a string. The skin of the individual to be vaccinated was incised and the string drawn through the incision. Alternatively cowpox scabs from a calf were

---

[45]National Archives, RG 94, Fort Churchill.
[46]Doten, *The Journals of Alfred Doten: 1849-1903*, 3 Vols., p. 951.
[47]Ibid., pp. 1069 and 1382.
[48]Lewis, *Martha and the Doctor*, p. 116.
[49]National Archives, RG 94, E 574.
[50]"Fort Douglas Medical History," Fort Douglas Museum, Salt Lake City.
[51]National Archives, RG 94, E 574.
[52]Ibid.

used for the vaccination. The frontier surgeon obtained the scab or "crust" in a vial from the medical purveyor, but quality control did not always produce an effective vaccine. Surgeon Lorenzo Hubbard in 1870 at Fort Bidwell ordered a second "crust" for vaccination because the first "crust" was ineffective.[53]

The vaccination to eliminate smallpox began in the eighteenth century, was reluctantly accepted in the nineteenth century, but was ardently applied by the frontier surgeon. The world-wide conquest of the disease continued until the late twentieth century when the infecting virus was removed from circulation. Today the virus only exists in laboratory cultures and health scientists debate the wisdom of killing these remaining specimens.

TUBERCULOSIS

While smallpox occurs suddenly and devastatingly, tuberculosis is insidious and causes a long, slow drain on the victim's health. Cases of tuberculosis were occasionally seen in the army, but generally the young soldiers were healthy. Private Green in March 1876 developed pulmonary consumption following typhoid fever and was discharged from the army by the surgeon at McDermit.[54] Surgeon Kober was more daring and decided to treat a patient he diagnosed as having tuberculosis.

Hammond, an emaciated new recruit with elevated temperature, a slight cough, and lassitude arrived at the base. Kober read in a journal that fresh blood was recommended for the treatment of consumption. (A Mormon home remedy in the 1800s also recommended fresh blood from a slaughter house for the treatment of tuberculosis.)[55] Since

---

[53]Ibid. Hubbard died at Fort Bidwell on Oct. 3, 1871, of chronic diarrhea.
[54]National Archives, RG 94, E 574.
[55]Fife, "Pioneer Mormon Remedies," p. 157.

soldiers at the post killed a steer every other day Kober induced young Hammond to drink a pint of beef blood immediately after the soldiers killed the animal. Records indicate that he regained his health in two months.[56] Unfortunately, they are imprecise as to how many treatments he took.

Doctors were also susceptible to tuberculosis and there are several records of Great Basin physicians who had the dreaded disease. Acting Assistant Surgeon George Munckton who served at Camp Nye in 1864, died of tuberculosis in San Francisco.[57] Later, a poignant and elegant clinical description of tuberculosis is given by Surgeon Vollum of his Fort Douglas assistant, Dr. John E. Spencer, who died of the disease.

> He inherited the disease from his father, developed it by overzeal in hospital and the dissecting-room, and he sought employment in the Army, with a view of getting stationed somewhere in the interior, elevated region of country, Circumstances brought him to this place. When he reported he was pale, thin, and feeble, having some time before had serious hœmoptisis; his pulse was small and rapid, and his respiration hurried and difficult, and a constant harassing cough, that brought up considerable expectoration, A walk of a thousand yards would require him to lie down to recover his wasted strength. His lungs were both consolidated at the top; there was a cavity of some size in the upper lobe of the left lung that gave out a rattling, sibilant sound that could be heard a short distance from him. The bracing weather of the fall coming on soon after his arrival. he commenced to practice a little horseback-riding, and before the winter was well advanced he could ride to Salt Lake City, three miles off, and back, with little fatigue, spending the remainder of the day in comparative quiet. By the following spring, though the winter was open, wet and changeable, the cavity in his lung was closed up, and gave out no sound to the ear on the chest, and tubular rales had mostly ceased, and his face took on the color

---

[56]Kober, *Reminiscences*, p. 270. This episode was also reported in *Greasewood Tablettes* 4, No. 2., 1993, p. 3.

[57]National Archives, RG 94, E 561, Munckton.

of health; he increased some twenty pounds in weight, and he expressed himself as being as well as he had ever been, his cough having subsided to a minimum condition of a hack, at long intervals, brought on by a bit of food, flying dust, or laughter. During this time he adopted no treatment whatever, and only occasionally took a glass of whisky as a tonic. Having occasion to go to Omaha a year and a half afterward, he contracted measles while there, and returned with his cough re-established and expectorating freely. The cavity in the left lung re-opened, and his general condition nearly as bad as it was when he first reported. Exposure at his door when half-dressed one night, to respond to a patient's call, gave him a chill that was followed the next day by nearly a fatal hœmoptisis. Fearing the influence of the coming winter, he took up his residence at Santa Barbara, Cal., and there regained the good condition he enjoyed at this place, but he allowed his energy to run away with him, he accepted two offices under the corporation, and, after an occasion of overwork and zeal connected with his duties, he had a hemorrhage and died.[58]

ALCOHOLISM

Alcoholism, always of concern on the lonely frontier and in boring distant military posts, occurred with regularity on the Great Basin frontier. Lieutenant Hein's comment about the men of his command at Fort Scott who "were nearly all addicted to drinking to excess" was not an exaggeration. In studying the drinking habits of certain classes of nineteenth-century citizens Rorabaugh stated that the "lustiest consumers of alcohol . . . shared one common trait: they were members of a new, mobile class without customs, roots, or social ties."[59] Furthermore, sociologists state that people drink to relieve anxiety.[60] These character traits certainly fit the miners, cowboys and soldiers of the newly settled Great Basin.

---

[58]*Circular No. 8,* p. 342. Hœmoptisis is a condition where hemorrhage occurs in the lungs and the individual coughs up blood. Tubular rales are noisy breath sounds caused by disease in the lungs.

[59]Rorabaugh, *The Alcoholic Republic: An American Tradition,* p. 140.

[60]Ibid., p. 146.

According to local oral history, the first death at Fort Bidwell occurred during an early winter when an inebriated soldier left the local saloon, jumped on his horse and headed south rather than north to the garrison. The next morning when he didn't show up for report a detachment from the garrison found wolves dragging his body toward the mountains where he had fallen off his horse and died from acute alcoholism and exposure.[61]

Doctors such as Corson at Fort Halleck also succumbed to this disease and bad habit. Since alcoholism was widely recognized as a problem, the military attempted to control the availability of alcohol around most Great Basin posts. In addition to the violence surrounding the excessive use of alcohol, withdrawal of alcohol could cause delirium tremens (DTs). This condition usually started after a drinking binge, an illness, or withdrawal from alcohol. It is characterized by a tremor, paranoid delusions and frequently coma or convulsions with swelling of the brain. When these later symptoms are present death is a threat. Between one and two percent of the admissions to Great Basin military hospitals carried the diagnosis of DTs. The treatment consisted of prescribing brandy or alcohol in diminishing doses in the hope that death could be prevented.

Once the DTs were controlled the soldier returned to duty. Alcohol rehabilitation or "taking the cure" was not a luxury afforded the soldier on-duty in a frontier fort. However, a popular cure for alcoholism at the time in Nevada was the Keeley Cure taken at Steamboat Springs, a resort midway between Carson City and Reno. Supervised by Dr. Simeon L. Lee, the treatment devised by Dr. L. E. Keeley who graduated from Rush Medical School included hypodermic doses of gold and NaCl (table salt). Keeley in 1880 revealed that the formula included "bichloride" or "Double

---

[61] Author's interview with Patricia A. Barry, May 15, 1994.

Chloride of Gold," but the total composition was never revealed. Unfortunately the cure was not any more effective than today's cure for alcoholism.[62]

VENEREAL DISEASE

Venereal disease—syphilis and gonorrhea—fluctuated in importance at the various forts. At the more isolated posts it was less of a problem than at bases located close to a town. Kober reported that at Fort Bidwell with a mean strength of forty-five to sixty-five during a twenty-three year period (1870-1893), there were only twenty-one cases of syphilis and during a seven year period (1886-1893) there were only eight cases of gonorrhea.[63] In contrast, at Fort McDermit with a mean strength of fifty-four to seventy-one men between 1870 and 1874 there were eighteen cases of syphilis and seven cases of gonorrhea.[64]

When soldiers at a base were infected the neighboring Indians became infected. Controls to prevent infection were marginally effective, but included: reporting of contacts with infected individuals so that treatment could be started earlier; educational programs for the soldiers; treatment of prostitutes; and licensure of brothels.

Treatment consisted of potassium iodide, but since this was not entirely satisfactory alternative methods were tried. When Native Americans and soldiers at Halleck became infected the doctor proposed curing the contaminated individuals with steam baths. The base commander ordered soldiers to construct lime and stone chambers over the hot springs at the nearby Myers Ranch. The "cure" consisted of steaming the genitalia while sitting over the springs.[65]

Venereal disease was more prevalent at Great Basin mili-

---

[62]Harris, *California's Medical Story*, p. 287, and Lender and Martin, *Drinking in America: A History*, p. 122.

[63]National Archives, RG 94, E 547, B 104, pp. 144-147.

[64]*Circular No. 8*, p, 514.

[65]Oral history by Earl Wright, recorded by Edna Patterson July 29, 1958.

tary bases toward the end of the century. At Fort Douglas in 1897 a "total of 123 men had VD from the 24th Infantry (colored) since their arrival . . ." The surgeon, Alfred C. Girard, proposed inspection of the prostitutes and the "keeper of the public house" agreed, but the city moved in and closed all of the houses. Girard continued, "Not for long, everything [the brothels] moved to 2nd West Street from Commercial Street (Regent Street)."[66]

During the frontier period, treatment for venereal disease was not always effective. Prevention and public health education, similar to modern times, were used by the military doctor in the Great Basin to curb the spread of syphilis and gonorrhea.

OPHTHALMIA

Ophthalmia was a common infection in the army, hence it was known as "Army Ophthalmia."[67] It was recognized in the Great Basin as a problem associated with the dry climate and dust. The soldier on the western frontier was living in constant dust while in the field. The powder-like alkali dust caused constant irritation. The eye irritation caused gray granulations associated with purulent exudate on the conjunctiva. It was contagious and sometimes epidemic. This is a classical description of trachoma that is caused by a microorganism, *Chlamydia trachomatis*. Trachoma is probably the leading cause of blindness in the world.

SCURVY

Scurvy was first recognized on long sea voyages during the sixteenth century, and in the eighteenth century James Lind (1716-1794), surgeon for the Royal Navy, described prevention of scurvy by inclusion of citrus fruits, now known to be rich in vitamin C. However, diets deficient in the vitamin

---

[66]"Fort Douglas Medical History," Fort Douglas Museum, Salt Lake City.

[67]Parkes, *A Manual of Practical Hygiene*, v. II, p. 153.

were the rule rather than the exception on the western frontier. The old adage, "Those who fail to study history are destined to repeat its errors," applies to Great Basin travelers and soldiers. Scurvy was a frequent visitor to the area, but it generally spared the Indian inhabitants who drank tea from plants rich in vitamin C.

In individuals with normal baseline levels of vitamin C, the period before signs and symptoms of scurvy appear is four to six months. Approximately three per cent of the stored vitamin C is used per day.[68] Most immigrants and soldiers probably had borderline levels of stored vitamin C and developed symptoms in less time. In 90 days fatigue becomes noticeable, after 130 days skin lesions appear, and the profound symptoms of edematous and bleeding gums with anemia and impaired hearing appear in 180 days.[69]

These symptoms in travelers from the east appeared about the time when they arrived at the Humboldt River in the Great Basin, four months away from civilization.[70] Scurvy was also a frequent visitor in the mining camps and western villages. In 1849, one fifth of the men at Sutter's Fort were on crutches and afflicted with symptoms of scurvy. One year later in the early mining camp of Sonora, Dr. Lewis C. Gunn of Philadelphia saw so many patients with scurvy that he credited the disease with establishing his reputation and practice.[71] Scurvy appeared sporadically at Fort Churchill, in the Oregon forts, and at Camp Three Forks, Idaho, when eating habits deteriorated, and fresh vegetables became unavailable.[72] Soldiers' life style and eating habits carried a risk of developing scurvy.

---

[68]Hodges, "Vitamin C," *Nutrition and the Adult: Micronutrients*, p. 75.

[69]Lorenz, "Scurvy in the Gold Rush," p. 474.

[70]Duffy, "Medicine in the West: An Historical Overview," p. 10.

[71]Lorenz, "Scurvy in the Gold Rush," pp. 475 and 491.

[72]*Circular No. 8*, p. xxxviii, and Record Group 94, Churchill Returns.

OTHER CAUSES OF DEATH

Local diseases as described by the surgeon general included respiratory illness and other inflammatory conditions. These and most of the other conditions described above rarely caused death. In many years there were no deaths, but when necessary the surgeons performed an autopsy to determine the cause of death. The first known autopsy in Nevada occurred at Fort Churchill when in 1862, Surgeon Furley determined that "Sergeant H. Auchenbach died very suddenly of Enlargement of the Heart without speaking to any one."[73] On April 29, 1869, Private Louis Phillippi died at Fort Halleck from "pneumatia metastasis & paralysis of the heart."[74] At Fort Halleck on May 17, 1874, an autopsy on William King revealed that he died from rupture of a liver abscess.[75] Acting Assistant Surgeon Frederick W. Elbrey in June 1874 at Fort Cameron stated that there was a death from peritonitis due to ligation of intestinal piles.[76] On April 20, 1881, Egan died of a ruptured aneurysm at Fort Bidwell.[77]

Other statistics from Great Basin posts revealed there were five deaths—one from fever, one consumption, two diarrhea and one homicide—at Fort Bidwell between 1870 and 1874.[78] During the same period at Fort Halleck there was one violent death.[79] At Fort Independence, Dr. Charles B. White reported one death from consumption during the four year period, and there were three deaths—one from

---

[73]National Archives, RG 92, Records of the Quartermaster General, Correspondence File, Fort Churchill. Nevada in this situation refers to the future state of Nevada.

[74]National Archives, RG 94, E 547, B 374.

[75]Ibid., B 376.

[76]Ibid., B 69. Intestinal piles usually referred to intestine prolapsed in a groin hernia. Ligation produced obstruction and certain death. Unfortunately some early surgeons did not recognize the true nature of the hernia and ligated the bowel.

[77]Ibid., B 101.

[78]*Circular No. 8*, p. 502.

[79]Ibid., p. 511.

diarrhea, one gunshot wound and one suicide—at Fort McDermit.[80]

These autopsies reveal that the doctor was able to find the diseased organ and the cause of death, but the doctor was not able to establish the cause of the enlarged heart, aortic aneurysm, pulmonary metastasis or liver abscess.

Forensic autopsies, when necessary, were also conducted by military surgeons during the era of frontier medicine. In 1886, One-Arm Jim, a Paiute who was acknowledged to be quarrelsome and dangerous, shot and killed Andy Kinnegar, a rancher and store keeper, during a robbery. Surgeon William P. Kendall at Fort McDermit performed the autopsy on the partially decomposed remains and testified that: "a track of a ball, either rifle or pistol, extending from the right nasal fauces of the deceased inward, downward and to the left, to a point over the seventh cervical vertebra, producing injury sufficient to cause death." One-Arm Jim became the first Indian in Humboldt County to be tried and sentenced for killing a white person. He died in the Nevada State Prison in Carson City in 1915.[81]

LIVING CONDITIONS AND PERSONAL HYGIENE

Up to this point, issues of health care—diseases and treatment—have been the primary focus, but it is important to look at living conditions as related to health. For living conditions such as housing and sleeping quarters and hygiene as related to food, dental hygiene, clothing, sanitation are important to health.

Sir John Pringle (1707-1782), a civilian who was Physician-in-Chief to British forces in Europe in the War of the Austrian Succession laid down the rules of personal hygiene

---

[80]Ibid., p. 514.

[81]The murder and trial was described extensively in *The Silver State* in 1886-87 and was researched by J. P. Marden of Winnemucca. Also see Rocha, "'Big Bill' Haywood and Humboldt County: The Making of a Revolutionary," p. 9.

in the eighteenth century: "adequate ventilation of barracks and hospital wards . . . proper clothing, avoidance of over-crowding . . . cleanliness . . . disposal of wastes, [and proper] construction of latrines."[82]

By the 1860s these principles were the "new wave" of therapeutic advancement in clinical medicine in the United States. Developed in France, empirical clinical observations resulted in de-emphasizing drugs with the promotion of nature's healing powers through the management of hygienic factors such as fresh air, exercise, cleanliness, and diet. Furthermore, the stress on hygiene lead to the development of public health and preventive medicine.

Supervision of hygiene was related to the health of the men in the regiment and was the responsibility of the surgeon. In the late 1800s many military physicians after they returned to civilian life, turned to teaching hygiene in the colleges and universities. After all, they had seen first hand the results of disease when hygienic measures breakdown in the command; when the water supply became contaminated; when food was tainted; and when epidemics emanated from the local sutler's store.

HOUSING

Housing for soldiers in the Great Basin was often crude and primitive. During the first winter at Fort Halleck the soldiers slept in dugouts and tents. In another example, Mrs. Orsemus Boyd and her officer husband spent their first two winters at Fort Halleck in a tent that didn't keep out the winter winds or rain.[83] Nearby at Camp Ruby, the conditions were not much better. The buildings were built of vertical logs placed in the ground resulting in structures that were little better than fenced corals with a roof.

---

[82]Bayne-Jones, *The Evolution of Preventive Medicine in the United States Army, 1607-1939*, pp. 10-11.

[83]Boyd, *Cavalry Life in Tent and Field*, pp. 30 and 78-79.

The sleeping arrangements were also poor. Men slept two abreast in a wooden bunk that was usually crawling with bedbugs. On July 12, 1870, the surgeon at Fort Halleck requested that the wooden bunks be replaced with metal bunks because it was impossible to eliminate the bugs.[84] Even so, seven years later, the surgeon officially reported to the district command that the poor state of health of the men at Halleck was due to the crowded condition of the living quarters.[85] This was also a problem at Fort Churchill which was considered to have one of the best living accommodations in the military district.

DIET

In a similar vein, providing sufficient and quality food was difficult in Great Basin forts. Inadequate and poor diet not only was a cause of conditions such as scurvy, but resistance to disease was decreased.

Soldiers sometimes existed for months on coffee, hard tack (a form of dried bread) and bacon—fresh vegetables were not available. For this reason, the post doctor at most western frontier forts planted a garden and more importantly, saw that the soldiers included vegetables in their diet. Assistant Surgeon Furley reported in 1852 from Fort Yuma, eighty miles north of the Gulf of California, that the principal diseases were diarrhea and scorbutus [from lack of vegetables].[86] At Fort Churchill he reported that the only vegetable available was the potato and noted that troops went for as long as four months without even potatoes. Raw potatoes were known to readily alleviate the symptoms of scurvy.

Besides contributing to poor health, the lack of roughage and fresh vegetables in the diet was a major factor in the cause

---

[84]Northeast Nevada Museum, Letters sent from Halleck.
[85]Ibid.
[86]Kober, *Reminiscences,* p. 142.

of constipation. Three percent of the admissions to Fort Churchill's hospital were for constipation. Fanny Corbusier commented that fruits and vegetables were rare at McDermit, but Native Americans brought dandelion leaves, mushrooms, wild garlic and onions to the post in the spring.[87] Her husband planted wild currants and roses on the base and established an irrigation system. The above fruits and vegetables have proven to be rich sources of vitamin C.

Although vegetables were necessary, meat was also important for troops on the move in the field against hostile tribes. At Fort Churchill, Furley noted that fresh beef although regularly available was "of such a leathery texture as almost to baffle the digestive power of anything but the stomach of an ostrich or a Soldier."[88]

Fort Halleck had similar problems with the quality of meat. First Lieutenant D. J. Craigie wrote to J. J. Campbell, the beef contractor, "It has been going from bad to worse & is now unfit to eat."[89] Even though beef was plentiful at Fort McDermit the quality was sometimes poor, and Corbusier raised pigeons and ducks. Fanny Corbusier noted the Indians killed blackbirds for food.[90] Two years later at Fort McDermit, Kober raised frogs for consumption.

Depending on the season, plenty of small game such as fish and prairie hens was available for food. Fanny noted the scarcity of large game was due to "Indians killing most of it." Most likely, then, as is now the case, the shortage of large game such as deer was due to winter kill from extreme weather. On occasion, food was scarce and Native Americans had a difficult time maintaining an adequate diet. At Fort McDermit, they collected the entrails from the slaughterhouse and

---

[87]Corbusier, *Verde to San Carlos,* pp. 98-99.

[88]National Archives, RG 92, *Churchill Returns.*

[89]Northeastern Nevada Museum, Letters from Halleck, May 22, 1877.

[90]Corbusier, *Verde to San Carlos*, pp. 93 and 98. Also see Kober, *Reminiscences,* p. 245.

took them to their camp for food. The various tribes in the Great Basin ate all parts of the cow. They even cooked off the hooves and used the remaining parts in vegetable stew. What they didn't eat they used for clothing and shelter.

Food was not always inadequate in the Great Basin. A typical meal for the men of Troop "C" of the 4th Cavalry at Fort Bidwell in 1893 was: Breakfast—hash, bread and coffee; Dinner—roast beef, boiled potatoes, beans, lettuce, bread pudding, bread and coffee; and Supper—cold beef, cold tomatoes, baked beans, bread and coffee.

When food preparation was good the morale was high, but when inadequate, morale suffered. Assistant Surgeon Washington Matthews reported in April 1874 at Fort Bidwell that the bread was bad because the substitute baker was inadequate. He noted the post cook was in the guard house for "intemperate habits." He was paroled and the bread improved. Matthews commented further, "This may not have been for the best interests of discipline; but unquestionably was for the best interests of digestion."[91]

DENTAL CARE

A good diet is not only necessary for good general health, but also for healthy teeth. Dental care in the military on the Great Basin frontier was primitive. For a toothache a soldier could expect little more than pain medication or extraction. Thus, in 1868 when Surgeon John C. Watkins at Fort Scott asked the Surgeon General to supply false teeth for an enlisted man the answer came back that the army does not provide teeth. Furthermore, the Surgeon General suggested that the soldier can only be sent to a local dentist if the soldier pays for the teeth. Continuing, he stated that if this is not possible and "the want of teeth renders him unfit for service he can be discharged."[92]

---

[91]National Archives, RG 94, E 547, B 104.
[92]National Archives, RG 94, E 561, 616.

In keeping with this policy, eight years earlier Assistant Surgeon Roberts Bartholow who was at Fort Crittenden received a temporary leave of absence to acquire false teeth. Bartholow contracted scorbutus while in Utah and a temporary set of upper teeth were "rendered useless" due to "the absorption of the alveolar processes." He received a thirty-day leave to find a dentist to fit him with "a permanent set of artificial teeth." Afterwards he returned to duty.[93]

CLOTHING

Even clothing was of poor quality and contributed to the low morale of the men. Reports from Fort Halleck on soldiers' garments in 1868 described the poor design and materials of the uniform. The pants were "coarse, ill-woven, loose material . . ." The seams were so poorly stitched that they only lasted one month. The "shirts were of fair material, but they were cut too low in the neck." The blouse was of inferior quality and the sleeves were too short. They soon wore out and the men were exposed to the elements. "Galling and blistering" of the feet due to the loose knit of the socks was a constant problem. Boot leather was of poor quality and soaked up water forcing the men to put extra leather or paper in their boots for protection. Their overcoats were poorly lined and made of poor quality cloth. The report, ending on a positive note, stated the blankets were "excellent, fine, soft, light and very warm. . . ."[94]

SANITATION

Of all the environmental conditions at the Great Basin forts sanitation and improper disposal of waste contributed the most to poor health. Yet, the importance of proper water supply and sewerage disposal was known for many years

---

[93]Ibid., Box 38.

[94]National Archives, RG 94, *Returns from Halleck,* and Patterson, *Sagebrush Doctors,* pp. 46-47.

before construction of the Great Basin forts. John Snow's work in the 1850s that showed cholera to be a water-borne disease was an important milestone.

The post surgeons were well aware of the water supply as a source for disease at Forts McDermit and Halleck. They pointed out that diarrhea resulted from filth draining into the water supply. Assistant Surgeon Charles B. Byrne in April 1872 recommended at Fort Warner drainage of the reservoir to remove the source of illness.[95] But out on the desert, water was scarce during the summer when the springs were low, increasing the chance for contamination. Then, water had to be transported in barrels. Needless to say, water for bathing was in short supply and cleanliness suffered, further increasing the risk of epidemic dysentery.

In addition to risk at the base, disease could be carried from the surrounding communities and ranches. The completion of the railroad through the Great Basin meant that the area was no longer isolated from epidemics in other parts of the country. As a result smallpox, cholera and scarlet fever were a risk at communities along the railroad. When outbreaks of epidemic disease occurred in Elko and other communities close to the bases the surgeon quarantined the post. He also exerted control over the local trading post when contagious disease resulted from poor sanitation at the post. On one occasion, the Fort Halleck surgeon had the floor of the sutler's store replaced because underlying filth was considered to be the cause of an outbreak of diarrhea at the base.[96]

Sanitation and hygiene go hand in hand. Poor ventilation and lighting in the barracks and other buildings on the post resulted in poor health and low morale of the men. Partly for this reason, new hospitals were built at Forts Halleck and McDermit. Even though new barracks were also constructed

---

[95]National Archives, RG 94, E 547, B 328.

[96]Patterson, *Sagebrush Doctors*, p. 52.

to improve ventilation and provide wash facilities, the men still had to bathe in nearby streams. Later, the soldiers dug irrigation ditches to improve the availability and convenience of fresh water. Nevertheless, at many times during the year when there was insufficient water for bathing the men suffered from lice in addition to bedbugs. The vermin proliferated in the hair of the men, in the straw mattresses and in the wooden bunks. Later, horse hair mattresses were provided and formaldehyde became available for disinfecting the sleeping quarters.

SURGICAL TREATMENT

A discussion of health care in the Great Basin would be incomplete without consideration of surgical treatment. Most surgery was minor and consisted of lancing abscesses and removal of foreign bodies, but on occasion, the surgeon had to perform an amputation or trephine the skull. Most surgery was performed to treat trauma or to treat life-threatening infection. Many of the military surgeons who practiced at a military base in the Great Basin had served in the Civil War and therefore had performed amputations on the battle field in primitive conditions and without anesthesia or asepsis.

Fortunately, although the conditions were primitive in the West, anesthesia in the form of chloroform and morphine was available. Asepsis or sterile technique was not used in the early period of military presence. As mentioned earlier this technique was introduced into the military in 1877, and it was introduced in civilian practice on the West Coast in 1879.[97]

AMPUTATION

Army surgeons utilized three methods of amputation: the circular, the oval and the flap operation. The simplest was the circular operation known today as the guillotine technique.

---

[97]Harris, *California's Medical Story*, p. 159.

After anesthesia and the application of a tourniquet, the surgeon made a circular incision around the entire circumference of the limb. The muscles were then divided superior to the skin incision with a circular sweep of the knife. The vessels were tied with silk suture. After retraction of the muscles the periosteum (the thin tissue covering of the bone) was incised and scraped with a rasp. Next, the surgeon sawed the bone above the muscle incision and then, smoothed the bone before closing the incision with silk. This quick—ten minute—circular technique was seldom used except for arm amputations. The disadvantages were: the skin scar was near the end of the bone and could result in ulceration due to deficient covering of the stump; and the stump was likely to become conical resulting in problems with a prosthesis.

The oval incision eliminated the problem of the scar being near the end of the bone, and was performed in a manner similar to the circular amputation. The only difference was that the incision was started higher on one side of the limb and finished at a lower level on the opposite side.[98]

Of the three techniques the flap method was preferred and variations of this method are used today. The physician could either make a long anterior or posterior flap, by performing a v-shaped incision on one side of the limb. The flap could include muscles or soft tissue in the flap or use skin alone. Inclusion of the muscles prolonged healing of the wound and therefore was seldom used. Teal's flap method consisted of a long, generally anterior flap and a short flap. The short was one fourth the length of the long. The breadth of the flaps was equal to one half the circumference of the limb.[99] In addition to amputations of the leg a modification of the flap method was used to amputate the arm, wrist and digits.

---

[98]Walsham, *Surgery its Theory and Practice*, pp. 632-34.
[99]Ibid., p. 634.

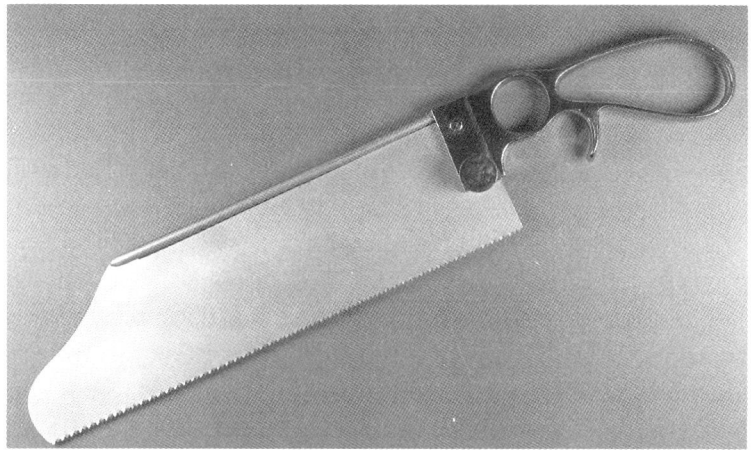

A Nineteenth Century Amputation Saw
Photograph by the author, University of Nevada School of Medicine Collection

TREPHINING

Surgeons performed trephination with a simple circular auger in situations where they diagnosed a simple closed fracture of the skull. Diagnosis was by palpation of the depressed fragment or the linear fractures. If the patient was unconscious anesthesia was not required. The procedure entailed removing a small plug of bone to relieve pressure and if necessary, evacuating the blood clot. Sometimes more than one core of bone was removed. Performed properly, the risk of death from the procedure was slight, but the risk of infection was high. During the Civil War trephination was performed on 220 cases with a mortality of 56.6 percent.[100] No information on the diagnoses is available for these cases and therefore they cannot be compared to Kober's five or six cases in which he had no deaths.[101]

---

[100]Kaufman, "Treatment of Head Injuries in the American Civil War," p. 844.

[101]Kober, *Reminiscences*, p.271.

SUMMARY

During the later years the best summary of diseases seen at the frontier forts is given by Kober for a sixteen-year period at Fort Bidwell. There were 1,307 soldiers with 1,648 cases of sickness and six deaths. Diarrhea accounted for 257 cases (15.6%); catarrhal infections were 249 (15.1%); rheumatism, 168 cases (10.2%); malaria, 135 cases (8.2%) which was brought in by the 2nd California Volunteers Cavalry from the Sacramento Valley; pneumonia, nine cases; five cases of tuberculosis; no typhoid fever; and no meningitis.[102]

Such a summary invites comparison with diseases of the American Indians and civilians in the territory. A determination of the prevalence of the various diseases in the civilian and Indian populations is difficult, if not impossible. First, there are no complete censuses and second, no attempt was made to record all illnesses other than patients seen at the Army hospital or listed in the local newspapers. Furthermore, there is a great disparity in numbers between military personnel, Native Americans and civilians. Not to be forgotten are the Chinese immigrants who formed a significant part of the civilian population. Their diseases were largely ignored.

In spite of these obstacles, it is interesting to compare hospital admissions in available records. Epidemics spread across all populations, military and non-military. It is also obvious that the risk for trauma—gunshot and accidents—was not just limited to soldiers. There are also differences that appear when the statistics of the military (Fort Churchill) and civilian (Saint Mary Louise) hospitals are compared.[103] (See Appendices IV and V.)

---

[102]Kober Manuscript, pp. 113-122.

[103]This comparison is for interest only and not statistical analysis since there are large discrepancies in the population—less than 500 individuals, mostly young males, lived at Fort Churchill versus approximately 13,500 people on the Comstock. There is also a 15-year time difference between Fort Churchill's admissions in 1860-1862 and Saint Mary Louise's in 1876-1877, and probably most important is the difference in classification of disease. Not to be discounted is Kober's observation that soldiers were more likely to be on sick call.

Intermittent fever (malaria) was clearly the most prevalent disease during the early military years accounting for 18.3 percent of admissions to Churchill's hospital whereas only 10.4 percent of the patients at Saint Mary Louise were related to "all fevers." This category included brain fever which was probably falciparum malaria and other forms of malaria. The decrease in malaria during the fifteen-year period might also be explained by the difference in years and the growing use and acceptance of quinine. In contrast, the civilian hospital had typhoid/typhus as the most prevalent disease with 18.2 percent.

At Saint Mary Louise, diarrhea and typhoid fever combined accounted for 21.6 percent of the patients compared to 11.6 percent at Fort Churchill. A good case could be made for better hygiene in the military where a surgeon oversaw the habits of the men, thus infectious diseases from contamination of the drinking supply would probably be less frequent.

Just 15 years earlier typhoid fever was not listed separately as a cause of diarrhea at Fort Churchill, but diarrhea was 11.6 percent. Military surgeons were probably more consistent in their diagnoses and were required to categorize them. The increased prominence of infectious gastro-intestinal disease could certainly partially be explained by the elimination of malaria as a threat and thereby producing a relative increase in other diseases. On the other hand, the diseases that produced diarrhea were well known through out the West.

Rheumatism or rheumatic fever was 4.4 percent on the Comstock and 10.9 at Fort Churchill. Close living quarters with several people sharing the side bed was common during the boom days on the Comstock, but the military also had several individuals sharing the same room. Due to these living conditions, the infectious sore throat associated with rheumatism would probably spread quickly among both groups.

Another notable difference between the two groups was the presence of tuberculosis in the civilian population and its absence in the military. Most recruits were screened for tuberculosis and eliminated from enlistment. On the other hand, mining is well known to be associated with dust inhalation and the increased threat of tuberculosis.

Burns were a threat in the mines; the Comstock was known for its subterranean hot water. Tunnel collapses, falls, and explosion injuries were weekly occurrences in the mines, while the soldiers had to contend with more missile wounds. An interesting future study would include the types of missile wounds, complications, morbidity, and mortality that were suffered by soldiers in the various wars in the Great Basin.

Another noteworthy comparison is the similar percentage of delirium tremens in both groups, military and civilian. Alcoholism was not diagnosed with any degree of accuracy on the frontier, but one of its major complications, delirium tremens, was not difficult to recognize.[104]

A review of admissions reveals nervous complaints, "nervous debility," as a frequent complaint at Saint Mary Louise. This disorder was seen solely in young female domestic workers, and accounted for 7.4 percent of the admissions. To understand the basis of the diagnosis one must study the socio-economic situation in the mining camps. On the other hand, psychological disorders were also described among soldiers, but they were probably under reported. Surgeon Kober noted psychological disorders among the American Indians. He witnessed the application of hot, dry stones on the umbilicus to treat hysteria.

There are also anecdotal accounts of a high prevalence of respiratory diseases among the Indians. The ranchers

---

[104]For certain all types of addiction were difficult to recognize. Narcotics and addicting drugs were available in drug stores and were added to various tonics and medicines.

believed this high incidence of pneumonia and pulmonary disease among the Native Americans was caused by their bathing in the springs during the cold weather.[105] There were also many accounts of viral epidemics such as measles and smallpox among the Indians living near the military bases.

In addition to noting the various diseases they experienced, Kober described some of the Northern Paiute practices at Fort Bidwell. They used internal and external herbs, dry cupping and scarification for some inflammatory conditions. The Indians treated rattlesnake bite with sucking, ligature and a poultice of chopped lupine.[106]

---

[105]Author's interview with Eugene Luckey May 17, 1994.
[106]Kober Manuscript, p. 213.

Non-military Activities of the Great Basin Army Surgeons

The primary duty of the military physician was to see to the health care of troops on duty in their jurisdiction. Even though, on occasion, they were at war with Native Americans, during epidemics and when needed the Army offered humanitarian help to neighboring Indian tribes. We have seen that soldiers accepted the responsibility of feeding and caring for those who lived near the fort, but what about civilians? Did all patients receive treatment at the posts in the Great Basin and did Army surgeons treat patients in surrounding communities? After Acting Assistant Surgeon John C. Watkins arrived at Camp Scott he wrote to the Department of California Surgeon General asking if he could practice outside the base. The reply read: ". . . Par. 1305 Rev. Reg. 1863 which requires that your whole time will be given to the public service. It is however, customary for Medical Officers to practice outside, and in fact, where, as in your case there is no Physician in the adjoining country, it is a matter of humanity, . . ."[1]

There were many instances recorded where doctors treated civilians at the post hospital. In August 1875 a run-away horse dragged a civilian named Carlton and he died forty-five minutes after arrival at the Fort Halleck hospital.[2] Also, railroad employees frequently visited the base and doctors treated them when they were sick or injured.[3] At Fort

[1] National Archives, RG 94, E 561 and see Appendix II
[2] National Archives, RG 94, E 547.
[3] Boyd, *Cavalry Life in Tent and Field*, pp. 78-79.

McDermit there were several references in the hospital ledger regarding civilian treatment and hospitalization. For example, in January 1875, O'Keefe, an indigent, was brought to the post with frost bite of the feet and received treatment.[4] At Fort Bidwell, frostbites were common among the citizens in the community and frequently a cause for amputation.[5] Entries in the hospital records of several Great Basin forts refer to frostbite and treatment by the base physician. Other diseases and injuries were treated in the post hospital.

In 1880, a citizen named "Franks," a Mexican, died in the post hospital of valvular heart disease.[6] Military hospital admission for civilians required consent of both the commanding officer and the post surgeon. Army regulations of 1874 permitted a charge for hospitalization up to $1.00 per day for civilians requiring food, nursing and medicine. The commander of Fort Bidwell allowed Kober to treat civilians at the base hospital for $1.25 a day with 75¢ going to the hospital fund, 25¢ for food, and 25¢ divided between the cook, nurse and steward.[7] As a result of the income from the hospital the surgeon usually became the post treasurer and used the hospital money to buy food and supplies.

In addition to hospital charges the surgeon could collect fees for his private service. Indigent patients received treatment without consideration of their inability to pay, but in some situations the base surgeon made enough to double his monthly pay. At Fort Grant, Arizona Territory, Corbusier's civilian practice only yielded $1,000 a year because the cattlemen were unable to pay. At other posts the post surgeon made four to five times this amount. The Indian Agency also paid the army surgeons for medical care.[8]

---

[4]National Archives, RG 94, E 547, B 410.

[5]Ibid., B 104.

[6]Ibid., B 411.

[7]Kober Manuscript, Box 19.

[8]Corbusier, *Recollections of her Life in the Army.*

The Native Americans at Fort McDermit were reluctant at first to use the white doctor's medicine, but when they lost confidence in their medicine men they accepted help. Five years after construction of the fort, three hundred Native Americans lived at the post. In January 1870 an epidemic struck; many were sick and several children died. Initially, they were "averse" to the military doctor's treatment, but the situation became desperate. In July they reconsidered and asked for treatment.

Also at Fort McDermit in 1874, two Paiute women were sick from poisoned vegetables; they were treated and recovered.[9] At Fort Bidwell in 1878, Matthews wrote in the hospital ledger about a similar situation: "A squaw living near the post was poisoned with 'wild parsnip.' She was unconscious and unable to swallow. Inhalation of ammonia almost immediately restored her to consciousness. The use of a stimulant and emetic rapidly cured her."[10]

At Camp Harney in 1871, Assistant Surgeon Charles B. Byrne noted that there were several cases of fatal tuberculosis among the Paiutes. In addition he recorded in the hospital ledger that during the winter months many were afflicted with bronchial diseases and diarrhea.[11] Other surgeons recorded the presence of pulmonary disease among the Indians. Careful records were also kept of the civilian patients.

In his autobiography, Kober carefully describes his civilian practice, pointing out that cowboys and shepherds contracted venereal disease more often than soldiers. The scarcity of the disease most likely was due to the remoteness of the base, since syphilis and gonorrhea were more prevalent at Fort Churchill which was close to the rowdy, brawling tent-cities of the Comstock. Nonetheless, the surgeon at Fort Churchill

---

[9]National Archives, RG 94, E 547, B 410.

[10]Ibid., B 104. Oral tradition in Patrica Barry's family at Fort Bidwell said that Indian women often used wild parship to commit suicide.

[11]Ibid., B 224.

in an eighteen-month period (1860-1861) treated only thirty-two cases of venereal disease (eighteen syphilis and fourteen gonorrhea).

Kober, further detailing his civilian practice at Fort McDermit. He opposed using instruments in childbirth and attending the labor of stockmen's wives within a radius of thirty-five miles.[12] On another occasion he treated "hysteria in an hypnotic form" in young women by inhalation of ammonia and instillation of a cold douche. Native Americans also had this disease and Kober was called by a "buck" to treat his wife who was "almost dead." When he arrived he found an old "medicine man" in the act of applying a heated knife over the pit of the stomach producing the desired effect.[13] He had another civilian case where a rancher sustained a ruptured spleen when kicked by a horse. Unfortunately, the patient had peritonitis on arrival at the post hospital and died shortly thereafter.[14]

At the conclusion of his tenure at Fort McDermit, Dr. Kober left the Great Basin in 1877 only to return in 1880 for duty at Fort Bidwell. For the next six years he was a contract physician at the fort and then, he pursued private practice in the community. While in private practice he was called on from time to time to "fill in" at the fort when a surgeon was sick or when there was a need.

When he arrived in 1880 the village of Fort Bidwell had two hundred inhabitants. Shortly thereafter, he helped develop two large cattle ranches, the Warner Valley Stock Company and the Lakeshore Cattle Company. In 1886 he brought his sister, Lizzie, to live in the community. He also brought to America two nephews, Henry and Karl. Their descendants live in California and Oregon, but none are left

---

[12]Kober, *Reminiscences*, p. 268.
[13]Ibid., p. 270.
[14]Ibid., p. 271.

in Surprise Valley. In an unpublished manuscript Dr. Kober describes the diseases and economics of practicing on the frontier.

There, Kober's outside practice netted fees that sometimes approached, but never exceeded $5,000 a year. He charged $3 a visit to patients within three miles of the fort and $1 a mile beyond the three mile radius. Obstetrical patients paid $25 for delivery as well as a mileage charge. In contrast the fees in Nevada fifteen years earlier were much higher. The first meeting of medical men in Nevada in 1872 set fees of $5 for a day visit, $10 for night visits, $10 per hour if detained, $100 for a manual delivery, $250 when instruments required, and $100 and up for surgery.[15] How faithfully the doctors adhered to this schedule is not known.

Kober saw a wide variety of diseases at Fort Bidwell. He documented them and kept accurate statistics. During his six years of practice at the town of Fort Bidwell, he saw a few mild cases of cholera infantum and one death from the disease, but cholera morbus was rare.[16] Although there were no cases of smallpox, measles affected "every family" in the spring of 1886. He treated over one hundred cases among the civilians without any mortality. On the other hand many Indians died from measles because they had no immunity to the virus.[17] Just as devastating for the ranchers in the area was scarlet fever.

In the spring of 1885, he saw twenty-four patients with scarlet fever.[18] In 1887 there were at least seven deaths from the dreaded sore throat that suffocated its victims. On February 2, 1887, the school was closed; February 10, the first death occurred, and the doctor recommended that there be

[15]Davis, *The History of Nevada*, p. 613.
[16]Kober Manuscript, p. 112.
[17]Ibid., pp. 113-114.
[18]Ibid., p. 114.

no public funeral because of the contagious nature of the disease. Scarlet fever spread though the community killing children with regularity until June. Dot Munroe wrote in her diary on May 17, 1887: "Poor Dr. Kober worked so hard and faithfully but it was no use."[19]

Diphtheria was even more deadly. Many cases appeared in April 1878 across the Warner Mountains near Alturas and there were many deaths. Kober saw one case in 1883 in the family of a farmer who built a home on the site of a corral "little suspecting that the excrementitious matter had for years permeated and polluted the soil, and thus prepared a hotbed for disease germs."[20] Diphtheria was eliminated by early diagnosis and antibiotics in the twentieth century, but croup, a viral disease that also suffocated infants was a threat in the 1880s. Kober honestly declared that he couldn't differentiate between diphtheria and croup.[21]

Mental illness was rare in Surprise Valley, but Kober described a case of religion melancholia with hallucinations and a case of hysteria in a male.[22] Tuberculosis was also rare. There was some glandular tuberculosis while in twelve years he saw only two cases of pulmonary tuberculosis among the five thousand settlers in the valley.[23]

Besides treating the patients in the vicinity of the base the surgeon could get help from other doctors in adjacent communities or even from remote cities. When Mrs. Biddle, the wife of an officer at Fort Halleck, was ill, Acting Assistant Surgeon Conant Brierly sent for Surgeon George Chismore from San Francisco. Chismore arrived and stayed by her side for two months. Eventually he sent her by train to San Fran-

---

[19]"The Diary of Dot Munroe—1886-1889," *J. Modoc Co. Hist. Soc.*, No. 10, 1988, pp. 30-48.

[20]Kober Manuscript, p. 115.

[21]Ibid., p. 117.

[22]Ibid., pp. 80-81.

[23]Ibid., p. 213.

cisco to complete her recovery.[24] Similarly, Dr. Loren Clark at Fort Halleck wrote the Assistant Adjutant General at the Presidio that "Mrs[.] Summerhayes is dangerously ill, and in so critical a condition that I desire a surgeon of experience to consult with."

The base military surgeon provided an important service to the surrounding community. Many times he was the only doctor available to civilians or Native Americans. A few remained in the community after their military service ended.

Besides taking care of patients the surgeons on the Great Basin desert had many leisure hours to pursue other activities. Game was plentiful in all parts of the Great Basin: deer were abundant especially in the mountain areas; antelope were found on the plateaus; duck and geese were found around the lakes; and sage hen were common. The soldiers and medical officers took advantage of the situation and hunted for recreation and food. At Fort McDermit, a favorite activity for the Corbusiers was horseback riding in the Santa Rosa Mountains.

Recreational activity aside, the military doctor was expected to be a competent scientific investigator. To further this activity the medical department supplied current literature so that the frontier surgeon could keep in touch with scientific advancement. Meteorology was conceived as a science in this country in the Army Medical Department.[25] All surgeons in the army and navy kept accurate data on the climate and the weather of the regions in which they served. Their records are recorded in "The Medical History of Posts."[26]

The West was considered to be a laboratory for natural history, geology, and anthropology. When a new frontier

---

[24]Biddle, *Reminiscences of a Soldier's Wife*, pp. 95-97.

[25]Busey, *Address to Graduates*, p. 9.

[26]*The Medical History of Posts*, National Archives Record Group 112, Entry 92.

post was established, the surgeon wrote a description of the flora and fauna in the surrounding desert, valleys and mountains.[27] Edward Perry Vollum became actively involved with describing the birds and their activities in the mountains around Fort Douglas. Like other frontier surgeons he sent specimens to the Smithsonian Institution. For his efforts he was recognized to be an outstanding ornithologist.[28]

Other Great Basin surgeons were more interested in anthropology and ethnology. In many areas the surgeon was the first educated person to have prolonged contact with the Indians. They learned their language, culture and provided detailed anthropological descriptions. Vollum, Kober, Corbusier, and Matthews were just a few of the physicians who wrote of their Indian neighbors. For their medical skills and scientific efforts they were respected by the native tribes. On more than one occasion they were spared the hostilities that were directed toward other intruders in the Great Basin.

Kober spent many of his leisure hours in Indian burial grounds collecting crania and skeletons. He found the bodies in shallow graves or covered with rocks and some, he noted, were mummified from the hot dry climate.[29] Kober shipped the crania to Rudolf Virchow, a leading figure in anthropology, and they are demonstrated on Plate xvi of his book, *Crania, Ethnica Americana Sammlung auserlesner Amerikanisher Schädeltypen.*[30] Corbusier, also, studied the Native American

---

[27]Surgeons at all of the Great Basin forts recorded scientific data of the vicinity of the post. In the spring of 1868 a large, leather bound book, entitled "Record of the Medical History of the Post," was issued to all "permanent" posts. Instructions specified that the first 80 pages were to be devoted to the natural history of the post, including botany, geology, etc. Each physician assigned to the base kept this record detailing the sanitary conditions and the health of the troops on a monthly basis. A summary of the reports from Forts Douglas, Three Forks, Warner, Harney, Bidwell, Independence, Halleck, McDermit, and Scott was published in 1870. *Circular No. 4.*, pp. 363, 428, 434, 436, 446, 450, 452, 453, and 454.

[28]Hume, *Ornithologists of the United States Army Medical Corps*, pp. 453-66.

[29]Kober, *Reminiscences*, p. 268. Virchow was also a physician and the father of pathology.

[30]Kober, *Reminiscences*, p. 226.

and later learned the Navajo language when stationed in the Arizona Territory, but at Fort McDermit he studied anthropology and shipped skulls to the newly established Army Medical Museum in Washington, D.C. Washington Matthews also shipped bones to the Army Medical Museum and became an expert on Native American culture.[31]

---

[31]Mattison, ed. "The Diary of Surgeon Washington Matthews, pp. 5-74.

Biographies of
Great Basin Military Surgeons'

William Hemple Arthur, born in Philadelphia on April 1, 1856, received his M. D. from the University of Maryland and then, studied chemistry for two years at Johns Hopkins. Like many military doctors at the turn of the century he served in the Indian wars, the Spanish-American War, the China Relief Expedition of 1900, the Philippine War and the First World War. In 1909 he became the first commander of the Walter Reed General Hospital and in 1915, the Commander of the Army Medical School. He retired as Brigadier-General in 1918 after thirty-seven years of service.[1]

Godfrey H. T. Ferdinand Axt was born in Germany November 24, 1835, and emigrated to New York where he enlisted as a private in the 20th New York Volunteers in May 1861. During the Civil War he became interested in medicine and was appointed Acting Hospital Steward. Axt participated in numerous battles including: White-Oak Swamp, Antietam, the first and second Fredericksburg and Chancellorsville. Without a medical diploma he was appointed Acting Assistant Surgeon U. S. Volunteers, May 1864. After the War, in 1866 he received a medical degree from University City of New York. In 1867 he traveled to California and accepted a position at Fort McDermit and received a commission. He retired from military service in 1870.[2]

Thomas Francis Azpell was born in Pennsylvania March 11, 1828. After graduating from Jefferson Medical College, in 1861 he joined the Army as a Surgeon for a volunteer unit from New Jersey. He served for four years in that capacity and received Brevet Lieutenant-Colonel for faithful and meritorious services. Rejoining the Army in 1867 at David's

---

[1]National Archives, RG 94, E 561.

[2]Henry, *Military Records of Civilian Appointments in the United States Army*, v I, p. 54; National Archives, RG 94, E 561; and *Directory of Deceased American Physicians*, p. 50.

Island, New York, he eventually traveled west and served at Fort Halleck in 1871. Azpell remained in the Army until 1885.[3]

Elisha Ingraham Baily was born in 1825 and graduated from Jefferson Medical College at the age of nineteen. He served in the Army in the West at Fort Floyd before the Civil War. After being there less than two months, he asked for transfer because the climate was not good for his health. Licensed in California in 1889, he died in San Francisco in 1908.[4]

Joseph C. Baily military record began in 1857 when he was appointed Assistant Surgeon from Pennsylvania. Previous to the military he graduated from Delaware College. His first field duty was at Fort Bridger, Utah Territory. While stationed there he served several short tours of duty at Fort Floyd, and had a relapse of intermittent fever. Baily accompanied Simpson while surveying the route from Salt Lake City to Carson City. During the Civil War he was in the Army of the Potomac and advanced to Surgeon. Returning west in 1865 he distinguished himself in Arizona and was Brevet Lieutenant-Colonel for faithful and meritorious services.[5]

John Henry Bartholf, born in 1830 in New Jersey, graduated from Columbia University College of Physicians and Surgeons in New York in 1854. During the Civil War he served as Assistant Surgeon of the New York Volunteers and was present at the battles of Fredericksburg and Salem Church. At the end of the War he was Brevet Captain for his meritorious service. Assigned to the West he served at Fort Harney for four years. After serving in the Army for many years he died in Washington, D.C. in 1918.[6]

Roberts Bartholow is best known as the first person to demonstrate electrical stimulation and localization of motor functions in the human brain. He was born in New Windsor, Maryland, on November 11, 1831. After receiving an AB from Calvert College he graduated from University of Maryland Medical College in 1852 and entered the Army in 1857. In 1858 he served a short tour of duty at Fort Floyd. He served in the Civil War, and in 1864 left the Army to settle in Cincinnati.

In 1869 he occupied the chair of materia media at the Medical College of Ohio. Bartholow started a journal, *The Clinic,* published several

[3]Henry, *Military Records,* p. 54, National Archives, RG 94, E 561, and RG 112, E 88.
[4]National Archives, RG 94, E 561 and *Directory of Deceased American Physicians,* p. 56.
[5]Henry, *Military Records,* p. 56 and National Archives, RG 94, E 561.
[6]Ibid., and *Directory of Deceased American Physicians,* p.82.

small books, wrote three prize essays, and wrote a book on pharmacology which sold over sixty thousand copies. While in Cincinnati he developed one of the best electrophysiologic treatment and research rooms in the country at Good Samaritan Hospital.

In 1874 Bartholow did the experiments demonstrating cerebral motor function in his laboratory which produced severe criticism from the medical community. A thirty-year-old feeble-minded patient had a rodent ulcer (basal cell carcinoma) of the scalp that exposed the cerebral hemispheres. Bartholow stated that the patient's "race was nearly run." With her consent and without anesthesia electrodes were inserted in the brain and electrical current applied. In addition to demonstrating motor function, convulsions resulted and the patient died several days later.

He became chairman of materia medica at Jefferson Medical College in Philadelphia in 1879 and remained a respected member of the faculty. He died in Philadelphia in 1904.[7]

Edwin Bentley was born in Connecticut in 1820 and graduated from the Medical Department of the University of New York in 1847. Appointed from his home state he served as Surgeon of the U. S. Volunteers for four and one half years during the Civil War and was Brevet Lieutenant-Colonel. While stationed at Fort Independence in 1876 he was admitted to the Napa Insane Asylum for three months. After his military service he moved to Arkansas where in died in Little Rock in 1912.[8]

William Cline Borden, the only son of a farmer preacher, taught school before he entered the medical profession as an apprentice in the office of a small town New York doctor. Four years later he entered Columbian Medical College (now George Washington Medical College). Upon graduation and after passing the Army Medical Board in New York City in 1883, he entered the United States Army at the age of twenty-five.

In 1887 during a three year stay at Fort Douglas, Lieutenant Borden made his first contribution to medical science. At the start of a lifelong interest in microscopy he published "An Extemporized Section Flattener," an article on cutting paraffin sections for examination by a microscope. This and later articles on the subject led to his election to the Royal Microscopical Society of London. Leaving Fort Douglas, Borden traveled the

---

[7]Morgan, "The First Reported Case of Electrical Stimulation of the Human Brain," pp. 51-64 and *Directory of Deceased American Physicians,* p. 82.

[8]Henry, *Military Records,* p. 57, *Directory of Deceased American Physicians,* p. 111, and National Archives, RG 94, E 561.

West for the Army. After the Spanish American War, he was assigned to Washington, D. C. where he published in 1899 a text on the "Use of the Roentgen Ray" that was printed by the Government Printing Office.

While in Washington he became friends with Walter Reed who researched the transmission of Yellow Fever. When Reed developed acute appendicitis Borden operated on him at Barracks Hospital (now Fort McMair). Reed died six days later. To commemorate his friend Borden labored for six years to establish the Walter Reed General Hospital which came to be known as Borden's dream.

After twenty-five years in the service, Lieutenant Colonel Borden retired with a heart condition and established a private practice in Washington. A year later in 1909, the President of George Washington University asked Dr. Borden to become dean of the medical school. His address to the District of Columbia Medical Society outlined the future direction of the medical school.

1. It is no longer possible to conduct an adequate medical school on a commercial basis.

2. A medical school should now be considered a school of applied science.

3. A medical school should be an integral part of a university.

4. A minimum entrance requirement of 4 years high school should be strictly enforced.

After twenty-one years as dean, a cerebral stroke forced his retirement in 1930. He died four years later.[9]

Edmund Gardner Bryant was a dashing, handsome doctor in early Downieville, California, and on the Comstock during the days of the bonanza strikes. From a prominent New England family and a cousin of Poet William Cullen Bryant, Edmund came west in a wagon train. A leading physician at the age of twenty-three in Downieville, he met and married sixteen-year-old Marie Louise Hungerford, the daughter of Colonel Daniel Hungerford. When the news of the massacre at Pyramid Lake reached the town in 1860, Bryant and Hungerford joined the California Volunteers and headed over the Sierra to join the defense of Virginia [City].

After the war his family joined him in 1863 and he opened a practice at Steamboat Springs in the new territory. Life in bars of the frontier city of Virginia was too much of a lure and he began to spend night after night

---

[9]Borden, "William Cline Borden 1858-1934," pp. 1-15.

away from home. In 1864 he disappeared and the family thought he went to San Francisco. The next they heard from him was in 1866 when they received word he was ill from alcoholism and drugs in a hovel near La Porte, California. Louise rushed to him and carried him on a litter to La Porte where he died June 20, 1866.

She returned to Virginia City where she later met and married John Mackay, one of the wealthiest men on the Comstock. John became the patron of the Mackay School of Mines at the University of Nevada. An early hospital in Virginia City, Saint Mary Louise Hospital, was named in honor of his wife, Louise.[10]

Samuel Franum Chapin was well known in California for his work in horticulture. Born in Otsego, New York, November 13, 1833, he grew up in Erie, Pennsylvania. Unable to attend college due to the lack of money he started the study of medicine in 1855 before attending medical school, but he eventually graduated from the University of Michigan Medical School and the Medical Institution of Yale College. During the Civil War he served with the Army of the Potomac at the battles of Williamsburg and The Wilderness.

After moving west he served as a contract civilian doctor at Forts McDermit and Churchill. Later, in California he practiced with Dr. Thorne in Auburn and in 1881 moved to San Jose. For several years he was State Inspector of Fruit Pests and a Director of the State Horticulture Society. Dr. Chapin, interested in fruit production, discovered the remedy for scale and issued important reports to fruit growers. On March 14, 1889, he was swept from his buggy and drowned while trying to cross a swollen stream in the Auburn Ravine.[11]

George Chismore became the most famous pioneer doctor in San Francisco and in the young state of California. Born in Ilion (Litchfield), New York, on January 1, 1840, he came west at the age of fourteen, to seek a new life in California. After working in the mining districts for six years and unhappy with his fortunes, in 1860 he began the study of medicine. Four years later he attended one term at the Medical College of the Pacific that was founded by Dr. Elias Samuel Cooper.

A northern adventure interrupted his studies when Chismore signed on as medical officer for the Western Union Telegraph Alaskan Expedi-

---

[10]Lewis, *Silver Kings*, pp. 72-73 and Berlin, *Silver Platter*, pp. 79, 96, 100, 111, 120, 124, and 128.

[11]The San Jose Historical Museum; San Jose *Daily Herald*, March 15, 1889, 2:5, and San Jose *Evening News*, March 15, 1889, 3:6.

tion. Returning to the States he signed a contract with the army in 1867. Colonel Charles Keeney, Chief Medical Officer of the Pacific, knew that Chismore had not graduated from medical school when he signed the contract.[12] During his five-year tour of service he spent two months temporary duty at Fort Halleck to take care of Mrs. Biddle, an officer's wife. Acting Assistant Surgeon Brierly realized Mrs. Biddle was dying and requested that Dr. Chismore be assigned to the case.

After his military service the thirty-three-year-old Chismore finished the course at the College of the Pacific in 1873 and then, practiced in San Francisco for thirty-three years. Early in his career he was also known as a "dentist and naturalist type physician." Chismore was president of the California Medical Society, twice president of the well-known Bohemian Club, chairman of the committee on genitourinary and dermatological disease for the medical society, chief surgeon of the California Women's Hospital, and president of the American Association of Genitourinary Surgeons. In 1881 he reported the first litholapaxy done in California. When he died in 1906 the *Examiner* hailed him as one of the greatest physicians in California. Flags in San Francisco flew at half-mast and a special train took his body to Santa Clara for interment.

The Bancroft Library in Berkeley has records of his Alaska expedition, journals of his many hunting trips, copies of his poems and writings on his opposition to homeopathy.[13]

William Henry Corbusier exemplified the qualities of the frontier doctor and army officer that were important in settling of the West. Typical of many of the doctors on the Nevada frontier, his first duty was preserving the Union during the Civil War. In 1864 at the age of twenty he volunteered and learned the skills of a surgeon on the battlefield. Leaving the army in June 1865, he went to medical school and graduated from Bellevue Hospital Medical College in New York City on March 1, 1867. Returning to his first love, military life, he signed on as a surgeon in the United States Army. Later, while stationed in Amite, Louisiana, he met and married Fanny Dunbar, a thirty-year-old school teacher. Before the wedding Corbusier traveled to New York to go before the Army Medical Board as a candidate for a commission, but the board had dissolved. He returned to Louisiana and his marriage took place while his mother-in-law "lay in her coffin in an adjoining room."

---

[12]Read and Mathes, *History of the San Francisco Medical Society*, v. 1, 1850-1900, p. 165.

[13]National Archives, RG 94, E 561; Holloway, *Medical Obituaries*, p. 84; Bancroft Library, *Chismore Journals*; and Harris, *California's Medical Story*, p. 231.

The newlyweds sailed to San Francisco where the young Dr. Corbusier started a practice, but the "damp, windy, and chilly" weather helped persuade them to accepted an offer to go to Camp McDermit. The pay was $125 per month including travel, housing, rations of food, fire wood and other provisions. They took the train to Winnemucca in July 1869 and rode by ambulance to the base where they served soldiers, Native Americans and ranchers for three "very happy" years. "We studied zoology, geography, French, history, etc., and gathered a great variety of beautiful wild flowers which we classified and pressed."

The Corbusier family left Nevada to serve in the Arizona Territory where they studied anthropology and the Southwest Indian culture. Responding to an appeal from the newly formed Army Museum, Corbusier sent skulls from tribal burial grounds. William Corbusier in 1876 passed the army examination and received a commission. His career choice sealed, he would remain in the army for thirty-two years. Reassigned to North Carolina, he received $1,600 a year, less money than he made while stationed in Arizona where, in addition to his $1,500 contract, he got $1,000 from the Indian Agency and money from private practice.

Typical of an army officer's family they moved frequently and traveled throughout the United States. At most stations he was able to make money on the side from civilian practice. His army career lasted until 1908 when he reached the mandatory retirement age of sixty-four. He had five sons, two of whom carried on the army tradition; one served in the army and another who was an acting assistant surgeon for eight years.[14]

Edward Evan Watts Corson had his career destroyed by a problem that was all too common in the military and in the West—alcoholism. Born March 16, 1848, in Pennsylvania, he studied at Tremout Seminary, Wyer's Military Academy, and Trappe School. In the spring of 1866 he trained in the office of Professor James A. Meigs, a faculty member of the Philadelphia College of Medicine. Two years later, after obtaining a diploma from the prestigious Jefferson Medical College he practiced three years in Philadelphia and attended the clinics at the Philadelphia Hospital.

In March 1873 Corson entered the U.S. Navy after passing the qualifying examination, but he was dismissed one year later because he was

---

[14]Corbusier, *Verde to San Carlos*, p. 3; Corbusier, *Recollections of her Life in the Army*. Record Group 94, Entry 561; and Coffman, *The Old Army*, p. 288 and 291.

"unfortunate enough to be reported to the department for being under the influence of intoxication drink on several special occasions. . . ." A letter from the navy recounted four incidents of Corson drunk on duty. Two were not proven but two led to a court martial where he was found guilty. When he applied for army service he wrote to the examination board, "I have reformed my habits." On 4 September 1874 he signed a contract for $125 per month and reported to Halleck.

A fire in Corson's building just one month after he arrived at his new assignment destroyed thirty texts, medical instruments and liquor. An inquiry by staff officers found him not negligent. Whether this incident was due to his problems with alcohol is not known, but certainly the suspicion is high. Less than six months later the army annulled his contract as a result of an incident involving the suicide of Lieutenant Alexander Grant on March 29, 1875.

Corson was the last person to see Grant alive and when called to the scene he was "under the influence of liquor, and in a stupefied [sic], dazed condition. . . ." Captain M. J. Stacey noted that Corson was reckless with the pistol and Stacy ordered him to his room with a guard. Captain Stacey wrote to headquarters requesting recall of the doctor, "I have the honor to request that it [the letter of recommendation for Corson] may be disregarded as the promises of reform given by this officer have not been kept."[15]

Frederick Denicke became interested in medicine in Germany where he was born. After immigrating to American, on January 7, 1863, he joined the 30th New York Volunteers as Assistant Surgeon and two years later received promotion to Surgeon. After the Civil War Denicke mustered out of the army and traveled west. Desiring a position as a surgeon in the Army, he wrote to the Department of California Surgeon General's Office stating that he had no diploma but had "passed successfully in surgery before a State Board of Examination in Hanover, Germany. I again successfully passed examination before a medical board at Albany, New York, in 1862."

As a civilian doctor he served at various forts until Fort Scott where he served from September 11, 1869, until February 22, 1871, when he was dismissed. He practiced in San Francisco until he died in 1883.[16]

William Eichelroth did not serve at a Great Basin military installa-

[15]National Archives, RG 94, E 561 and 574. Also Letters from Halleck at the Northeast Nevada Museum.

[16]National Archives, RG 94, E 561.

tion but did serve with the army at the Pyramid Lake battle where he was wounded in the nose when his horse was shot. He is also famous for the duel he fought with the editor of the *Aurora Times* over a dog. The duel took place with each combatant straddling the state line to prevent interference from the law. Neither participant was seriously injured but Eichelroth chipped a piece of bone from his antagonist shin.

Eichelroth, born in 1824 in Saxony, studied medicine at Jena and immigrated to New Orleans in 1849. For fourteen years he wandered the Mother Lode District mining and practicing medicine part-time. From 1860 until 1866 he ranged from Carson City to Aurora, Nevada, and finally decided to return to St. Louis to practice. During the moving preparation he lost his baggage and as a result decided to stay in the West. After settling in Sonoma, California, he was chief of the Tuolume County Hospital for many years and served in the California Assembly. He died in 1896 six years after retiring from practice.[17]

Charles Carroll Furley, born March 17, 1838, in New Jersey, came west with his family in 1850. His father, destitute, came to start a new life in his profession as a jeweler. Young Charles helped a man who collapsed on the street and in gratitude was given a set of medical instruments to help him on his way to become a doctor. He graduated from the recently formed Cooper Medical College in San Francisco in 1860.

At the start of the Civil War Furley enlisted in the cavalry of the Second California Volunteers as Assistant Surgeon and served two years, including one year at Churchill. He relieved Assistant Surgeon Milhau and became the second doctor to be stationed at a fort in the Western Great Basin. While at the fort he contracted and wrote about ophthalmia, a condition he was to suffer from for the rest of his life. In 1863 he resigned from the Army and traveled the Orient for one year as physician for the Pacific Mail Steamship Company. Returning to the United States he rejoined the Army and served as a surgeon in the Army of the Potomac until the end of the Civil War. After one year in Wyoming and a brief sojourn to Abilene, Kansas, he moved to Wichita in 1871, where he spent the rest of his life.

In the new community Furley presented a commanding presence with a dignified and scholarly attitude. Contributing to medical journals, he wrote about his experience in preventing childbirth infections by the use of cold water sitz baths. As a member of the Episcopal church, a staunch

---

[17]Dunlop, *Doctors of the American Frontier*, pp. 117-18; and Harris, *California's Medical Story*, p. 381.

Republican and Odd Fellow he was highly visible in community affairs. Furley was instrumental in starting the Wichita Library in 1876. Also active in professional organizations, he was member of the American Medical Association and a delegate to its convention in 1878. He was President of the Kansas State Society in 1878 and 1879 and helped found the South Kansas Medical Society becoming its first president. Furley was instrumental in founding the short-lived Wichita Medical College, which collapsed due to lack of students and funds.

Toward the end of the century the town of Wichita was threatened from lack of railway connections with Chicago. Furley and a group of business leaders stepped forward and formed the Omaha, Abilene and Wichita Railway Company. To insure its success they elected Furley president. He responded by developing the town of Furley on the new railroad. The last seven years of his life he was Treasurer of the Board of Education of Wichita schools. Charles Furley, a respected early citizen of Wichita, died in 1902 from tuberculosis.[18]

John Charles Handy lived perilously and was described by Judge Sloan in Tucson as "a man of strong will, aggressive, and both quarrelsome and vindictive."[19] He was one of the most colorful physicians to serve at a western Great Basin military installation. Born in Newark, New Jersey, on October 20, 1844, Handy came west at the age of nine with his family and pursued his medical education in San Francisco. Dr. Elias Samuel Cooper, the most important physician in early California, was Handy's mentor when he commenced studying materia medica at the age of fifteen. Cooper allowed the best opportunity for operative surgery because he "had control of surgery of this state through his fame. . . . I took up the study of anatomy procuring material for dissection in the vicinity of this city [San Francisco] during which time I had several narrow escapes from detection."[20] His training consisted of studying ten hours a day for three months and attending four courses of lectures.

After his medical education he tried private practice for three years. He relates "the only incident in my career that I look upon with regret was the death of a child I operated upon for hydrocephalus which might have been avoided if I had not operated."[21]

---

[18]*Pacific Medical and Surgical Journal,* 7 (June 1873), p. 183, and Jones, *The Medical and Business Career of Dr. Charles Carroll Furley.*

[19]Cosulich, *Tucson,* p. 138.

[20]National Archives, RG 94, E 561.

[21]Ibid.

Handy did not graduate from medical school, but was a volunteer doctor from California during the Civil War. On October 3, 1864, at the age of twenty, he took the qualifying examination for the army, but did not pass. In 1867 he served as a contract doctor at Fort McGarry for eight months. He requested that his contract be annulled. The Arizona Territory was more appealing than the desolate, dreary Nevada post. He left the state and traveled to the Southwest where he became the leading doctor in Tucson.

His career in the Arizona Territory began at Fort Thomas. Handy became embroiled in an extended argument with the post trader, Aaron Hewey, and fatally wounded him. A written note from the dying Hewey was entered into evidence at the trial stating that Dr. Handy was not to blame for the shooting. As a result Handy was exonerated.

In later years, Mr. Samuel Hughes, "the father of Tucson," related how the doctor came to establish practice in Tucson. In "about 1874" Dr. John Handy was in Tucson to find suitable homes for three orphan Native American girls, having personally escorted them in order to alleviate their fears. Handy spoke fluent Apache and was a trusted friend and considered a powerful medicine man. Hughes, who had moved to Tucson years previously, was seriously ill with lung hemorrhages and summoned Handy. Impressed with the handsome young doctor's skills and manner, Hughes inquired as to what would entice him to settle in the city. Handy replied that if he had an annual income of $2,500 he would stay and open an office. Hughes immediately found twenty-five families who would each guarantee $100 a year to have the services of the talented doctor.[22]

Dr. Handy's skill and reputation grew throughout the territory and he became the most prominent doctor in the community. As the County Physician he treated jail inmates and the indigent along with his more wealthy patients. However, his forward and outspoken manner continued to get him into conflicts. He spoke out publicly and in court against other physicians with whom he did not agree or when he thought they misdiagnosed a case. In addition, "his aggressive personality and vindictive spirit made him enemies."[23] On the other hand his civic awareness and responsibility were beyond question. Serving on the Board of Health and Board of Supervisors, his dedication to the community was recog-

---

[22]Whitmore, "Arizona's Pioneers in Medicine."

[23]Cammack, "A Faithful Account of the Life and Death of Doctor John Charles Handy," pp. 36-39.

nized and in 1886 he was chosen to be on the Board of Regents and appointed the first Chancellor of the newly planned university. Again, problems developed and he was dismissed from the board. Dr. Handy, also was at odds with city officials who were trying to clean up the streets. They closed the sewer line from his house that was dumping raw sewerage into the street and he responded with a law suit.[24]

His marriage was also disintegrating and the frequent fights were aired in public. To make matters worse Mary, his wife, became addicted to morphine prescribed by him. Dr. Handy filed for divorce and physically threatened any attorney who would represent his wife. His day of reckoning came when Frank Heney, an attorney who had a grudge with the doctor, took the case. A fight broke out and a shot silenced the loud argument at the corner of Church and Pennington streets in Tucson. At noon on September 24, 1891, Handy stumbled to his office mortally wounded. The next day he died. Flags flew at half mast and the body was sent by train to Oakland in the Bay Area where Handy had started his career in medicine. In spite of Heney's ulterior motive, the jury found the defendant not guilty. Perhaps they recalled the earlier shooting where Handy was the winner in a similar shooting.[25]

Henry S. Haskins reported to Halleck in May 1873 as an acting assistant surgeon. Initially, because of a deformed leg the army questioned his ability to perform medical and other functions at an army base, but a friend wrote in his behalf and stated that his problem did not cause him disability or prevent him from performing his duties. He remained at Halleck until October 1874. From there he went to Fort Bidwell and then served at various posts as an acting assistant surgeon until 1902; a career of thirty years as a contract doctor.[26]

William Pratt Kendall, born on September 10, 1858, in Pittsfield, Massachusetts, graduated in 1882 from Columbia Medical College in New York City. He started his medical career in the Army in 1885 when commissioned a First Lieutenant. He served four years at Fort McDermit, and on June 15, 1889, he closed the hospital and became the last military doctor to serve in Nevada during the frontier days. After his service at Fort McDermit he advanced to the rank of Captain. He retired in 1916 as a Colonel.[27]

Charles A. Kirkpatrick was born in 1823 in Missouri and spent his boyhood years on a farm in Illinois. At the age of sixteen he "became a

[24]Karolevitz, *Doctors of the Old West*, p.77.

[25]National Archives, RG 94, E 561.   [26]Ibid.   [27]Ibid.

Christian" and left home to become a missionary. One year later he returned to his father's farm. In 1841 Kirkpatrick enrolled in the first class at Knox Manual Labor College where he received a teaching certificate. In 1848 after attending lectures at the Medical College of Ohio, he opened practice in Grafton, Illinois. A short time later caught in "whirlpool of excitement" he left for California.

Keeping a diary on his trip west he described his brief sojourn in St. Louis where he had a picture taken of his "likeness." He was convinced that "virtue did not visit there." In March and April, 1849, he helped organize a wagon train of fifteen wagons, signed on as doctor and headed across the Missouri River.

His diary describes the trials and tribulations on the trail, but he fails to recount his medical experiences other than when he was so sick that he rode in the wagon for ten days. On September 3 they stopped at Donner's "Cannibal Camp" and Kirkpatrick took a souvenir tooth from a skull. (The Donner party camped near the site of the future town of Truckee, California, in the winter of 1946-47.) January 27, 1850, found Dr. Kirkpatrick in the placer mines of the Sierra Nevada.

Typical of the pioneer western doctor, Kirkpatrick moved freely from community to community seeking his fortune. In 1859 he was postmaster and physician in Benicia. He wrote in *Hutching's California Magazine*, June 1860, about the decline of salmon fishing on the Sacramento River as the result of placer and hydraulic mining. However, there were more important things on the horizon with the start of the Civil War.

Volunteers were mustered in from the Mother Lode and in 1861 Charles joined a California volunteer unit consisting of seven companies of soldiers bound for the Nevada Territory. They passed through Forts Churchill and Halleck before arriving in the Ruby Valley during a snow storm in September. He and his unit built Fort Ruby. One of the four Kirkpatrick children, an infant daughter died at Ruby. After a year at the log fort Kirkpatrick was ordered to Fort Douglas in Utah. He returned to California where he remaining in the army until March, 1866.

The family moved to Redwood City, the home of his wife, where he opened his practice. In 1871 Kirkpatrick obtained his Medical Degree from the University of California. For the remaining twenty-one years of his life he raised a family and was a leading citizen in Redwood City. He headed a committee to collect money for the victims of the Chicago fire and had the first sidewalk in town.[28]

---

[28]Researched by Mrs. Nita Spangler of Redwood City, California, and see the Kirkpatrick Diary Manuscript in the Bancroft Library.

George Martin Kober was one of the leading medical educators in the United States after he left the military. Born March 28, 1850, in Alsfeld, Hessen-Darmstadt [Germany], at the age of sixteen he emigrated to America to join his brother and sister. The 1848 revolution in his homeland convinced his father that his sons should not serve in an army under a German King. Young George, sparked by an interest in medicine and the knowledge that in Germany barbers were surgical assistants, became an apprentice in a barber shop. As was the custom, he moved in with the family, but in the New World surgery had already moved away from the barber shop. After a short stint as a barber he joined the army to become a hospital steward and pursue his dream. On a temporary duty trip to Chicago, Kober had an attack of pneumonia. His treatment consisted of a saline cathartic, dry or wet cupping or a mustard plaster, followed by a diaphoretic, ammonia acetate and spirits of nitre. The theory was to remove the toxins through the kidneys and skin by use of these drugs.

Having compiled an excellent record, Kober was ordered to the Surgeon General's office in the Ford Theater in Washington, D.C. In 1871 he went to Georgetown University Medical School located next door. The course lasted from 5 PM to 10 PM and the anatomy laboratory opened at midnight. He graduated in 1873 and volunteered July 1, 1874, to be a contract surgeon in the Pacific region.

After a short stay at Fort Alcatraz in San Francisco he was ordered to Fort McDermit in Nevada. Before he left San Francisco he indicated to a friend that he would rather stay in the more exciting Bay Area. With the intent of making a career in the army, he took the Army medical examination and failed. His most important duty was at Fort Bidwell where he also had a large private practice.

Leaving the army in 1886, he traveled for two years and then settled at Georgetown University. Initially appointed to a position in hygiene, he became Dean of Georgetown Medical School in 1901. He was dean, a member of the board of trustees, and led the school when it became a leading medical institution. During his life time he wrote 200 articles including his first, *Urinology and its Practical Applications*, published while stationed at Fort McDermit. He retired as dean in 1928.[29]

Washington Matthews was recognized for his knowledge of ethnology and philology of Native Americans. Born in Ireland in July 1843, the son of a doctor, Matthews graduated from the University of Iowa Med-

---

[29]National Archives, RG 94, E 561, and manuscript file at the Nat. Lib. Med.

ical Department in 1864. He entered the army and served until the end of the Civil War. A few months later he rejoined the army to pursue his scientific interests.

From 1865 until 1871 he studied the languages and culture of the Arickaree, Hidatsa and Mandan of the Upper Missouri River Valley. He wrote *Grammar and Dictionary of the Hidatsa* (1873), *Hidatsa English Dictionary* (1874), and *Ethnography and Philology of the Hidstsa Indians* (1877). The following five years Matthews was stationed in Nevada, California, and the Northwest. His stay at Fort McDermit was less than a month; he was then stationed at Fort Independence in the Owens Valley and later at Fort Bidwell.

After duty in the Museum and Library of Surgeon General's office he accompanied an archeological expedition to the Southwest. In 1893 he published *The Human Bones of the Hemenway Collection (1893)*. Later, he wrote *Navaho Silversmith* (1883), *The Mountain Chant: A Navaho Ceremony* (1871), *Navaho Legends* (1897), and *The Night Chant* (1902).

Matthews retired from the army as a major in 1895 and died ten years later in Washington, D.C.[30]

John Jefferson Milhau, a Frenchman, came to the Nevada desert in June 1860 at the time of the Pyramid Lake war. Commissioned in 1851, he served at various forts throughout the West. During this period he pursed his interest in anthropology and ethnology. While stationed at Fort Umpqua, Oregon Territory, Dr. Milhau wrote reports to the Smithsonian about the religion, language, living conditions, canoes, and physical appearances of the Umpqua and Coos Indians.

Four years later he was ordered to Fort Churchill, but he left after one month and went east where he distinguished himself during the Civil War. Promoted to major in May 1862, he was Brevet Lieutenant Colonel in 1864 for gallant service during the campaign before Richmond, Virginia, and in March 1865 became a Colonel for gallant and meritorious service during the war. After the war, another promotion to Brigadier General resulted from meritorious and distinguished service at Harts Island, New York, where a cholera threatened the community. He resigned his commission in 1876 and died fifteen years later.[31]

---

[30]Mattison, ed., "The Diary of Surgeon Washington Matthews, Fort Rice, D. T.," pp. 5-74.

[31]Beckham, "Lonely Outpost: The Army's Fort Umpqua," p. 247; Beckham, *Land of the Umpqua: A History of Douglas County, Oregon*, pp. 158 and 177; and National Archives, RG 94, E 561.

William Morrow Notson at the age of twenty-two graduated from Jefferson Medical College in his native city of Philadelphia in 1858. He was wounded in the Battle of Gettysburg and received two brevet promotions for meritorious services during the Civil War. After the war he was stationed at the future site of Fort Concho on the west Texas frontier. At the base he wrote "a moving, rich account about life and the struggle to build a pioneer society in a land devoid of luxuries."[32] Like all early frontier surgeons his duty included recording meteorology and describing the flora and fauna in the vicinity of the fort. From November 1874 to December 1877 he served at Fort Douglas in the Wasatch Mountains. Seven years later, after promotion to the rank of major, he died at the Columbus Barracks in Ohio.

James Lycurgus Ord's father, James Ord, was a son of King George III of England by his morganatic marriage to Marie Anne Frizherbent. Through such an agreement the heirs, although legitimate, cannot ascend to the throne. James Lycurgus, born May 18, 1823, raised in Washington, D.C., attended Georgetown College and graduated from Jefferson Medical College in 1840. Seven years later he joined the United States Army as a contract surgeon and sailed to Monterey with troops to occupy California. Lieutenants Henry W. Halleck and William Tecumseh Sherman were members of the party.

For a period of forty-five years Dr. Ord served in the military at different forts, including Fort Halleck, named after his sailing companion. He also served in the army during the Civil War and the Mexican War. In 1870, he was vice president of the California State Medical Society and chairman of the reorganization committee. By 1882 Ord was the United States Minister at Mexico City. After briefly settling in Santa Barbara he married the wealthy widow of Manuel Jimeno Casarin, an early pioneer and land owner, and became Collector of the Port.

The Ord family was staunchly military. Dr. Ord's father was an officer in the American Army during the War of 1812 and his grandfather, Captain Cresap, erected Fort Cresap near Washington to defend the settlement against hostile Indians. Three of his brothers, one being the well-known General E. O. C. Ord of Fort Ord fame, were officers during the Civil War and three of his nephews were officers in the army. His only daughter married an officer in the army. James L. Ord died October 3, 1898, and is buried in Arlington Cemetery.[33]

---

[32]Notson, *Fort Concho Medical History January, 1869 to July, 1872*.

[33]Santa Barbara Historical Society; *California Pioneer Register and Index 1542-1848*; and *Los Angles Examiner*, November 14, 1905.

Robert Maitland O'Reilly, born in Philadelphia, January 14, 1845, served in the army as a medical cadet at the end of the Civil War. Returning home he graduated from the University of Pennsylvania Medical College in 1866. He entered the army as a contract surgeon and after passing the examination by the Army Medical Board received a commission. Two years later he spent nine months (October 1869-June 1870) as a first lieutenant at Fort Halleck. He was chief surgeon during the Sioux expedition in Upper Arizona before returning east for tours of duty.

During the Spanish War he served with distinction and after returning to the states had several important appointments including chief surgeon of the Department of California. During that assignment he became Surgeon General of the United States Army (1902-09).

O'Reilly's most important contribution while Surgeon General was the reorganization of the medical corps. He took the first steps to eliminate the terms, "assistant surgeon" and "surgeon," and also proposed substituting "Reserve Corps of Medical Officers" for the unpopular title of "contract surgeon." Another noteworthy activity was his collaboration with Major William C. Borden on the subject of military surgery in W. W. Keen's *American Textbook of Surgery* (1903).[34]

Adrian Suydam Polhemus, born on January 3, 1856, at Astoria on Long Island, New York, grew up in a respected family originally from the Netherlands. He graduated from Phillips Academy in Andover, Massachusetts, and attended Yale College. The summer before he graduated from Yale he took "the ordinary tour of Europe parading mostly on foot with a small party of classmates and Harvard men." After graduating he studied in the office of Professor James R. Wood and received his degree from Bellevue Hospital Medical College in 1882. He describes the first year in medical school as "devoted largely to dissecting and laboratory work in histology and chemistry."

In July 1883 after medical school he entered the army as a contract physician. He passed the Army examination. From 1883 until 1886 he served in Nevada at Forts Scott, McDermit and Halleck. His career was interrupted in 1895 because of drug addiction. After a leave he returned and remained in the army until 1904 when he retired as a major.[35]

Benjamin Franklin Pope was born February 24, 1843, and raised in

---

[34]National Archives, RG 94, E 561, RG 112, E 88, Phalen, *Chiefs of the Medical Department United States Army 1775-1940*, pp. 79-83, and Pilcher, *The Surgeon Generals of the Army of the United States of America*, p. 91.

[35]National Archives, RG 94, E 561.

Rome, New York. He had attended Hamilton College in Oneida County, New York, for two years when the Civil War started. He tried to enlist but was rejected because he was, in his words a, "slender half-grown boy." He then studied medicine under his father, graduated from Albany Medical College and attended clinical courses at Bellevue Hospital Medical College in New York City. After completing his studies he entered the Army July 18, 1864, as an assistant surgeon in the 10th New York Artillery, which was a unit in the Army of the Potomac. Mustered out of the military in July 1865, he continued his clinical studies. Pope tried private practice before joining the Army and serving at Fort Halleck. In 1878 he took the Army examination and qualified as a commissioned officer. Serving until 1902, Colonel Pope died of chronic interstitial nephritis in the Philippines.[36]

Robert King Reid was born in Erie, Pennsylvania, on January 21, 1820. At the age of twenty-two he graduated from Jefferson Medical college and later, received a post-graduate degree from the University of Pennsylvania. After a short stint in private practice in South Carolina, like so many other young physicians he caught "gold fever." Electing to take the faster way to the gold fields he sailed south, traveled across Panama and up the coast to California. Shortly after arriving in 1849 he established a small practice on the Mokelumne River in a mining camp.

Dr. Reid became interested in psychiatry. He was the first superintendent of the California State Hospital, the first exclusively psychiatric hospital west of the Missouri River. In 1856, two years after he married the matron of the hospital, he lost his position as a result of a change of administration in the state house. Traveling to Paris, Reid continued his studies in the European clinics. Back in California in 1860, he established a practice in Stockton, but a short time later he enlisted as a California Volunteer in the Civil War.

During the War he was a surgeon in Stockton's Third Infantry Volunteer Regiment. For five years, including tours at Forts Ruby and Douglas, he served with distinction in the Union Army rising to the rank of colonel by "coolness, gallantry, and skill. . . . His record describes the situation. On January 1, 1863, 150 miles north of Salt Lake City, he was engaged in a battle for four hours against hostile Indians. Killed were 224 Indians and 15 soldiers; six soldiers later died of their wounds.

While her husband was busy as a volunteer surgeon during the Civil

---

[36]Ibid.

War Mrs. Reid prospected in the mountains around Fort Douglas. In 1863 she discovered and filed claim on a silver vein in Brigham Canyon. The canyon became the largest copper mine in the West.[37]

After the Civil War he returned to private practice in Stockton where he became a leading physician in the community. He was also a Vice-President of the first California State Medical Society. He died on February 4, 1891.[38]

Bernard Gustavus Semig, born in Pesth, Hungary, on April 27, 1840, graduated from the University of Vienna on Easter, 1863. After traveling to England and then to the United States he joined the army as a steward, but served only a short time. He enlisted in the Navy and sailed to San Francisco where he joined the army as a contract surgeon in 1866. Semig was wounded on April 26, 1873, in the Modoc War while giving assistance to a wounded soldier. He was wounded in the shoulder and neck and while disabled he sustained a wound in the left foot which resulted in amputation. In October 1874 he returned to duty, and then served at Camp Halleck for one month in 1876 and later, for one year at Fort McDermit.[39]

Charles Smart, born September 18, 1841, in Aberdeen, Scotland, was educated at the University of Aberdeen. Attracted by the Civil War, he came to America where he immediately joined the 63rd New York Volunteers and the Army of the Potomac. After examination by the Army Medical Board he was commissioned first lieutenant. He served in the Battle of Richmond where he was brevetted to the rank of captain for "meritorious service in the field during the campaign." In 1876 he was stationed in the Great Basin at Fort Douglas.

Because of his intellect and dedication he had many important assignments. He was a member of the National Board of Health and supervised the division on Sanitation and Statistics in the Surgeon General's Office. Perhaps Smart's most important work was on the medical history of the Civil War. In 1888 he edited the concluding volume of *The Medical and*

[37]Woyske, "Women and Mining in the Old West," p. 38, and *The War of the Rebellion*, Series I–v. L–In Two Parts, Part II–Correspondence, Etc., p. 318.

[38]Ibid.; Holloway, *Medical Obituaries: American Physicians' Biographical Notices in Selected Medical Journals Before 1907*, p. 378; Rogers, *Soldiers of the Overland*, p. 15; Thompson and West, *History of San Joaquin County*, p. 141; *Medical Society State of California*, 1891, v. 21, pp. 320-321, and Brody, "Hospitalization of the Mentally Ill during California's Early Years: 1849-1853," and Harris, *California's Medical Story*, p.152.

[39]National Archives, RG 94, E 561. Also see *Surgeon General's Report to Congress, 1883*.

Surgical History of the War of the Rebellion.[40] He also organized the Hospital Corps of the U. S. Army. In addition to numerous professional articles on military medicine and sanitation, he published a novel, *Driven from the Path*, (New York: Appleton & Company, 1872).

When the Army Medical School was established in 1893, Dr. Smart was appointed Professor of military hygiene. He retired with the rank of brigadier general in 1905 and died three months later in Saint Augustine, Florida.[41]

Alonzo Francis Steigers was born in St. Louis and graduated from St. Louis Medical College. He became an acting assistant surgeon in the Army after his medical studies were completed.[42] In January 1871 while he was with a scouting party, an Apache shot him in the left shoulder and the bullet exited at the wrist. A surgeon amputated his arm above the elbow.[43] The army declared him disabled, but the Secretary of War intervened, allowing him to continue his military service. He served in the military from 1865 until 1892 and spent sixteen months at Fort McDermit from June 1883 to October 1884.[44]

Anton William Tjader, born in Russia in 1825, received his medical education at the Royal Scandinavian Institute in Sweden. During the Crimean War (1854) he served in the Russian Army as a surgeon. At the age of thirty, he immigrated to American and entered Harvard Medical College, graduating two years later. Between 1857 and 1859 he served as a captain in the Navy at the United States Marine Hospital in Massachusetts and briefly as a contract surgeon in the Army.

After his brief military service he traveled west. In Nebraska he sustained wounds during an Indian battle. North of Salt Lake City he treated patients wounded during an Indian raid. After arriving at Genoa, Utah Territory, near Carson City, he became involved in community affairs, established a medical practice, and staked a mining claim. He had been in the territory less than one year when he took part in the Pyramid Lake battle, where he once again was wounded.

In 1861 Tjader was appointed Official Surgeon to the Nevada Militia.

---

[40]Henry, *The Armed Forces Institute of Pathology: Its First Century 1862-1962,* p 89.

[41]Kober, *Reminiscences of George Martin Kober, M.D., LL.D.*, pp. 215-218, and National Archives, RG 94, E 516, Boxes 529-530.

[42]National Archives, RG 94, E 561.

[43]*The Weekly Arizona Miner*, 14 Jan. 1871. p. 3.

[44]National Archives, RG 94, E 561.

One year later he married Lucy Curry, the daughter of Abe Curry, one of Carson City's founders. When he died in 1870 from the lingering effects of Indian arrow wounds, his widow was left with two infant sons.[45]

Edward Perry Vollum, born September 11, 1827, in New York City, became a recognized ornithologist of the U. S. Army Medical corps. After graduating from Jefferson Medical College he was appointed Acting Assistant Surgeon in May 1853 at the rate of $40 a month. Two weeks later he passed the entrance examination and was commissioned Assistant Surgeon. During his career Vollum served at many posts across the western frontier. Dr. Vollum was eager to respond to a request from the Assistant Secretary of the Smithsonian for specimens. He sent specimens of birds, skins, nests, fossils, and eggs to the Smithsonian Institution. His collection and correspondence are part of the Institution's permanent collection.

Vollum also helped Henry Sibley build the prototype tent copied from the western Indians that became known as the "Silbey tent." After its popularity was assured—the tent was used extensively by the North and South during the Civil War—Silbey reneged on his promise to share the discovery with Surgeon Vollum.[46]

At the start of the Civil War, Vollum was recalled from duty in California to Washington, where he served in the Army of the Potomac. During the war he was a participant in the battles of the second Manassas (Bull Run), Sharpsburg (Antietam), Gettysburg, Lookout Mountain and Missionary Ridge, Red River (Arkansas), and Mobile Bay. His primary duties included Medical Inspector, but he was also responsible for obtaining medical supplies for several armies in the field.

After the war his duties took him back to the West where he served against the Shoshones in Utah while stationed at Fort Douglas. During that period he catalogued the birds of Salt Lake City and continued his correspondence and shipping of specimens to Professor Spencer Fullerton Baird of the Smithsonian.

Colonel Vollum died in Munich, Germany, in 1902. His ashes are interred in the National Cemetery at Arlington, Virginia. The principal street that approached the Fort Douglas hospital was named in his honor.[47]

---

[45]His biography was thoroughly researched by his great-great grandson, Gary N. Tjader of Los Altos, CA.

[46]Johnson, "Taking a page from the canny Comanche, Henry Sibley devised a new tent for the Western frontier," p. 8.

[47]Hume, *Ornithologists of the United States Army Medical Corps*, pp. 453-66.

John C. Watkins from Whately, Massachusetts, remained an acting assistant surgeon because he was thirty-two, four years over the age limit, when he requested to take the examination for a commission.[48] He served eleven months at Scott from May 1868 to April 1869. When he needed assistance in the hospital he asked for a steward to be assigned to his post and received an answer that he could appoint one.

Charles Braman White was born in Vermont in 1826 and died of sarcoma August 10, 1881. His autobiography as told in a letter to the United States Army Medical Department tells the story of his life.

> I was born at Thilford Vermont on the 14th of February 1826. My parents were of the old N. England stock, my mother being from the Ellsworth of Conn. and my father a descendant of William White of the Mayflower.
>
> In 1828 my parents removed to the state of New York, to the village of Osewego, Tioga Co., and remained there till 1841 when my father being appointed president of Wabash College they removed to Crawfordsville, Indiana.
>
> I entered Wabash College in 1842 and was graduated there at in 1846. I spent the next academically year at the seminary of Andover, Mass.
>
> My Health failed in the fall of 1847 and returning home to [illegible] in the summer of 1848 I began the study of medicine. I went south in the fall and continued my studies under the preceptorship of Dr. Anson Brackett of Gainsville, Alabama.
>
> I attended medical lectures during the winter of 1850 and /51 and 1851/52 at the Medical Department of the University of Louisiana and received the degree of M.D. "pro minitis" in March 1852. In July 1851 I received the degree of A.M. from Alma Mater.
>
> I practiced medicine in the summer of 1851 in the county of Madison, Miss., being advised and encouraged thereto by Dr. V. H. Fugate of Miss. who recommended me to the people of the neighborhood which was in his immediate vicinity.
>
> I commenced practice in N. Orleans in 1852 and have continued there in practice ever since.
>
> For seven years I was physician to an orphan Asylum of the city and lost my position Jan 1st/63 because of my well known attachment to the U.S. government.
>
> I was visiting physician to the Charity Hospital of N. Orleans for two years. This is not a position of honor or emolument. It gives opportunity to [illegible] experience. After the battle of Shiloh I went to Corinth and came back in charge of wounded soldiers.

---

[48]National Archives, RG 94, E 561.

The arrival of the U.S. Fleet in N. O. soon after, was opportune for me as I had not taken the oath of allegiance to the confederacy, and detectives were already looking up "traitors." Prison, a confederate prison, certainly, perhaps, expulsion to Miss. without a pass, which amounted to hanging to the first tree out of the lines, was my expectation, but the Stars & Stripes came soon enough to save me, and many others.

I saw the secession flag of Louisiana hoisted with firing of cannon; I saw it come down in defeat and shame, and the flag of my fathers and of my country float in its place—God Save the flag.

From Jan 19 to June 30th, 1863, I was in charge of wards in U.S. Genl. Marine Hospital as acting assist. Surg. U. S. A. with the patients under my care during a portion of that time.

I was ordered to Baton Rouge immediately after the 1st assault upon Post Hudson for temporary duty, and by acting Med Director Van Norstrand assigned to the organization of Harney House branch Hospital. After 20 days since at B Rouge closed my connection with the government with the month of June.

I was married in Oct 1852 and buried my wife among her kindred in the "hill country" of Conn, July 11t, 1863.

My practice of my profession has been always legitimate, according to the obligations of my degree.

/s/Charles Braman White[49]

Alfred Woodhull graduated from Castleton Medical College in Vermont and joined the army at the start of the Civil War. He attended Lee's surrender at Appomattox with General Ord and later, served four months at Fort Halleck. During his final years in the army he taught hygiene at Princeton. He published the work, *Military Hygiene for Officers of the Line*, (NY: John Wiley & Sons, 1909), that became the standard in the military. He received a LL.D. from Princeton and lectured at Princeton on hygiene. His honors included the Gold Medallist of the Military Service Institute in 1885 and the Seaman First Prize in 1907 for teaching hygiene at a military school.[50]

---

[49]Ibid.

[50]*U. S. Army Surgeon General's Office Autobiographical Sketches of Medical Officers*, Nat. Lib. Med., MS C44.

Data on Great Basin Military Physicians

FORT BIDWELL

NAME	DATE/BIDWELL	POSITION	EDUCATION
Benjamin, George Arenfed[1]	Oct. '71-Mar. '72	Contract Surgeon	Transylvania Med Coll, Lexington, Ky
Bentley, Edwin	Feb.'77	Assistant Surgeon	Med Dept U of NY
Caldwell, Daniel G.	Sept. '69-Sept. '70	Assistant Surgeon	Unknown
Dods, William B.	July '66-Oct. '69	Contract Surgeon	Unknown
Fisher, Walter W. R	Nov. '86-Jan. '88	Assistant Surgeon	U of N.Y.
Handy, John C.	Dec. '65-May '66	Surgeon, California Volunteer	Cooper Med Coll (San Francisco)
Haskins, Henry S.	Nov. '74-Oct. '77	Contract Surgeon	U of Mich
Horn, George H.	July '65	Assistant Surgeon, California Volunteer	Unknown
Hubbard, Lorenzo	Aug. '70-Oct. '71 Died	Contract Surgeon	Bellevue Hosp Med Coll (NYC)
Kent, Lewis A.	May '82-July '82	Contract Surgeon	Unknown
Kober, George Martin	Jun. '80-Nov. '86 Dec. '87-Feb. '88 June '93-Oct. '93	Contract Surgeon	Med Dept George-town Coll, (Wash DC)
Kollock, Matthew H.	Jul. '66	Contract Surgeon	Unknown[2]
Matthews, Washington	Nov. '77-July '80	Assistant Surgeon	State U of Iowa Med Coll
Orr, Samuel Little	Sept. '73-Oct. '74	Contract Surgeon	Unknown
Patterson, William H.[3]	March '72-Oct. '73	Contract Surgeon	Unknown
Raymond, Henry Ingle	Feb. '88-Nov. '89	Assistant Surgeon	Unknown
Stirling Frank S.	May '66-Sept. '66	Contract Surgeon	Cooper Med Coll (San Francisco)
Todd, David Byron	June '78-Sept. '78	Contract Surgeon	U of Mich
Wakeman, William James	Nov. '89-May '93	Assistant Surgeon	Unknown

[1] Information regarding name, dates, fort, position and education is from the National Archives, RG 94, E 561; *Directory of Deceased American Physicians, 1804-1929*; and Butler, *The Medical Register and Directory of the United States*, unless otherwise noted.

[2] In 1888 Kollock applied for admission to New York Homeopathy Medical College.

[3] Patterson founded the Patterson Ranch in Surprise Valley.

FORT CAMERON

NAME	DATE/CAMERON	POSITION	EDUCATION
Cooper, James F.	Sept. '76-Oct. '76	Contract Surgeon	Unknown
Cowdrey, Stevens G.	Dec. '77-Sept. '81	Assistant Surgeon	Berkshire Med Coll, Mass.
Elbrey, Frederick W.	June '72-Sept. '74	Contract Surgeon	Coll Phy Surg NY
Notson, William Morrow	Nov. '74-Dec. '77	Assistant Surgeon	Jefferson Med Coll (Philadelphia)
O'Callaghan, Edward J.	Jan. '74-Jan. '75	Contract Surgeon	Unknown
Robertson, John J.	Sept. '81-Dec. '81	Contract Surgeon	Unknown
Snively, David S.	May '72-June '72[4]	Contract Surgeon	Unknown
Strong, Norton	Dec.'81-June '83	Assistant Surgeon	Chicago Med Coll

FORT CHURCHILL

NAME	DATE/CURCHILL	POSITION	EDUCATION
Benn, John E.	June '66-Aug. '66	Contract Surgeon	Unknown
Brierly, Conant Bowdin	July '69	Contract Surgeon	Toland Med Coll (San Francisco)[5]
Brown, Isaac W.	Feb. '63-July '63	Assistant Surgeon, First Lieutenant, California Volunteer[6]	Unknown
Burns, John E.	May '66-Aug. '66	Contract Surgeon	Cooper Med Coll (San Francisco)[7]
Chapin, Samuel Farnum	Aug. '65	Contract Surgeon	Coll Phys Surg (NYC)[8]
Ensign, William H.	Aug. '66-July '67	Contract Surgeon	Unknown
Furley, Charles Carroll	Nov. '61-Dec. '62	Assistant Surgeon	Cooper Med Coll (San Francisco)[9]

---

[4]Camped near Beaver.

[5]Harris, *California's Medical Story,* pp. 134-5. Toland Medical College, started by Dr. Hubert H. Toland in 1864 became the University of California Medical School in 1873. Brierly who graduated in 1866 became a University of California graduate. Also see Fort Halleck regarding Brierly's service.

[6]Brown was a volunteer assistant surgeon in the 3rd Battalion Mountaineers of California. See *Roster of Regimental Surgeons and Assistant Surgeons in the U.S. Army Medical Department During the Civil War,* p. 2. Also see Fort Ruby regarding Brown's service.

[7]Burns is listed in National Archives, M 617 as an acting assistant surgeon, but he is not in medical personnel file 561. Also see Harris, *California's Medical Story,* pp. 131-4. Dr. Elias Samuel Cooper organized the first medical school in California in 1858 by obtaining a charter from the University of the Pacific, a Methodist school in San Jose. Cooper's school was chartered as the Medical Department of the University of the Pacific.

[8]*Medical Directory of the Pacific Coast, 1880-1881.* Also see Fort McDermit regarding Chapin's service.

[9]*Directory of Deceased American Physicians,* p. 543. Furley was a member of the 2nd Cavalry of the California Volunteers.

Harrison, John T.[10]	Nov. '68-July '69	Contract Surgeon	Unknown
Hartsuff, Albert	Nov. '67 & Nov. '68	Assistant Surgeon, Captain	Castleton Med Coll (Vt)[11]
Mechem, Abel F.	Oct. '64-July '66	Contract Surgeon &Assistant Surgeon, First Lieutenant	U of Md[12]
Milhau, John Jefferson	June '60-Oct. '61	Assistant Surgeon, First Lieutenant	Coll Phys Surg (NYC)[13]
Ramatka, F. A.	July '67-Dec. '67	Contract Surgeon[14]	Unknown
Steele, Walcott	July '63-Oct. '63	Assistant Surgeon, First Lieutenant[15]	Unknown
Vansant, John	July '61-Nov. '61	Assistant Surgeon, First Lieutenant	Jefferson Med Coll (Philadelphia)[16]
Willson, John	Oct. '63-Sept. '64	Assistant Surgeon, First Lieutenant[17]	Unknown

FORT CRITTENDEN

NAME	DATE/CRITTENDEN	POSITION	EDUCATION
Baily, Elisha Ingraham	July '58-Aug. '58	Assistant Surgeon	Jefferson Med Coll (Philadelphia)
Baily, Joseph C.	Aug. '58-May '59 Aug. '59-Oct. '59 Jan. '60-May '60	Assistant Surgeon	Unknown
Bartholow, Roberts	Aug. '58	Assistant Surgeon	U of Md
Brewer, Charles	Aug. '58-Apr. '59 June '50-May '60 Sept. '60-Oct. '60	Assistant Surgeon	Unknown
Clements, Bennett Augustine	Sept. 58-July '59 Aug. '59-May '60	Assistant Surgeon	Nat Med Coll, (Wash DC)
Covey, Edward N.	Aug. '58-Feb. '59 Oct. '59-May '60	Assistant Surgeon	U of Md
Cuvier, John M.[18]	Dec. '58	Assistant Surgeon	Unknown

---

[10]See Forts Halleck and Ruby regarding Harrison's service.

[11]National Archives, RG 112, E 88. Also see Forts Ruby and Scott regarding Hartsuff's service.

[12]Holloway, *Medical Obituaries*, p. 307.

[13]Ibid., p. 311.

[14]Ramatke is listed in National Archives, M 617 and in RG 94, E 561, but the folder is missing.

[15]Steele entered the Nevada 1st Cavalry as a volunteer assistant surgeon during the Civil War. He is the only volunteer doctor listed from Nevada. See *Roster of Regimental Surgeons and Assistant Surgeons*, p. 109.

[16]National Archives, RG 112, E88.

[17]Willson is listed in National Archives, M 617 and in Smith, Jr., "The Sagebrush Soldiers," p. 39. There is an announcement of the First Annual Ball [Fort Churchill], February 22, 1864, The invitation committee was Willson of Fort Churchill and National Guard Surg. Gen. Tjader of Carson City. Also see *Virginia Evening Bulletin* 1864.

[18]Langley, ed., *To Utah With the Dragoons*, p. 128.

Getty, Thomas	Aug. '58-Jan. '59 Mar. '59-May '59 July '59-May '60	Assistant Surgeon	Pupil, Wm Harris of Philadelphia
Moore, John	Aug. '58-Aug. '59 Oct. '59-June '60 Oct. '60-Sept. '61	Assistant Surgeon	Pupil, Wm van Buney, Bloom- ington, Ind.
Norris, Basil	Sept. '58-Sept. '59 Oct. '59-May '60	Assistant Surgeon	U of Pa (Philadel- phia)
Porter, John Bliss	Aug. '59-Sept. '61	Surgeon, Med Director Dept of Utah July '59-Sept. '61	Unknown
Ridgely, Aquila Talbott	May '58-June '59	Assistant Surgeon	Unknown
Ryland, Kirtley	Jan. 58	Assistant Surgeon	Unknown
Williams, Thomas H.	Sept. '58-Sept. '59	Assistant Surgeon	Unknown

Fort Douglas

NAME	DATE/DOUGLAS	POSITION	EDUCATION
Arthur, William Hemple	Oct. '83-April '86	Assistant Surgeon	U of Md
Birmingham, Henry P.	Jan. '99-Nov. '99	Assistant Surgeon, Volunteer	Unknown
Borden, William Cline	May '84-June '86	Contract Surgeon, Later, commissioned	George Washington University (Wash DC)
Brown, Isaac W.	June '63	Assistant Surgeon, California Volunteer	Unknown
Burroughs, Charles L.	Mar. '75-Oct. '75	Contract Surgeon	Rush Med Coll (Chicago)
Cannan, John J.	Oct. '98-Nov. '99	Contract Surgeon	Unknown
Chapin, Alonzo R.	June '83-Nov. '83 Feb. '84-April '84	Contract Surgeon and Assistant Surgeon	Unknown
Clements, Bennett Augustine	Nov. '77-Sept. '79	Surgeon	Nat Med Coll, (Wash DC)
Deshon (De Shon), George Durfee	Dec. '94-Jan. '95, Mar. '95-Nov. '96	Assistant Surgeon, First Lieutenant	Bellevue Hosp Med Coll (NYC)[19]
Edie, Guy L.	Sept. '88-May '91	Assistant Surgeon	Unknown
Girard, Alfred C.	Nov. '95-April '98	Surgeon, Major	U of Würtzburg
Hamilton, John F.	Mar '66-Oct. '67	Contract Surgeon	Unknown
Heizmann, Charles L.	Oct. '91-Oct. '95	Surgeon, Major	Unknown
Horton, Samuel Miller	April '80-Oct. '83	Surgeon	Unknown
Johnson, Richard W.	Oct. '97-Nov. '97	Assistant Surgeon, Captain	Unknown
Kendall, William Pratt	March '91 June '91-Oct. '95	Assistant Surgeon	Columbia U Med Coll (NYC)
Kirkpatrick, Charles A.	Oct. '62	Assistant Surgeon, California volunteer	U of Calif (San Francisco)

---

[19]*Directory of Deceased American Physicians.*

Kirkpatrick, Thomas J.	Nov. '96-April '98	Assistant Surgeon. First Lieutenant	Unknown
LeCompte, Edward Palmer	May '78-Aug. '78, Nov. '78-May '80	Contract Surgeon	Mo Med Coll[20]
Meachem, Frank	Dec. '67-June '69	Assistant Surgeon	Berkshire Med Coll, Mass.
McPhaill, Benjamin Grisby	Nov. '75-June '76 Aug. '77-Oct. '77	Contract Surgeon	Med Coll of Va
Murray, Francis X.	Oct. '82-May '83	Contract Surgeon	Unknown
Niles, Harry Dorr	June '98-Jan. '99	Contract Surgeon	Unknown
Penrose, George Hoffman	May '98-June '98	Contract Surgeon	U of Buffalo Med Dept
Polhemus, Adrian S.	June '93-April '96	Assistant Surgeon	Unknown
Potter, Samuel Otway L	Feb. '83-June '83	Contract Surgeon	Jefferson Med Coll (Philadelphia)
Richards, George R.	Dec. '65-Feb. '66	Assistant Surgeon, Michigan Volunteer	Unknown
Reid, Robert King	Oct. '64[21]	Surgeon	Jefferson Med Coll & U of Pa, (Philadelphia)
Robinson, J. King[22]	Dec. '64-June '65	Assistant Surgeon, California Volunteer and Contract Surgeon	Unknown
Schutz, Edwin George	Oct. '98, Nov. '98-March '99	Contract Surgeon	Unknown
Smart, Charles	July '76-Dec. '77	Assistant Surgeon	United U of Aberdeen, Scotland
Smith, Andrew Kingsbury	March '66	Surgeon	Jefferson Med Coll (Philadelphia)
Spencer, John E.	Sept. '71-Feb. '73	Contract Surgeon	Unknown
Spencer, William C.	June '69-Oct. '70	Assistant Surgeon	Unknown
Steele, Walcott	Jan. '63	Assistant Surgeon, First Lieutenant	Unknown
Strong, Norton	Aug. '80-Dec. '81, May '83-Oct. '83[23]	Assistant Surgeon	Chicago Med Coll
Taylor, Hugh L.	Oct. 99-1900-	Contract Surgeon	U of Denver Med Dept
Thayer, Benjamin F.	Nov. 65-June '66	Contract Surgeon	Unknown
Vollum, Edward Perry	Aug. '70-Aug. '76	Surgeon	Jefferson Med Coll (Philadelphia)
Wakeman, William James	Sept. '82-Oct. 82	Assistant Surgeon	Unknown
Ware, Isaac Palmer	June '92-July '92	Assistant Surgeon	Bellevue Hosp Med Coll (NYC)

---

[20]Ibid.

[21]Orton, *Records of California Men in the War of the Rebellion, 1861 to 1867,* p. 197 and 522.

[22]After leaving the Army in 1865, Robinson entered private practice in Salt Lake City. He erected buildings with the intent of establishing a hospital near a hot mineral springs north of the city. His murder on October 22, 1866, was a result of conflict with the Mormons over the use of the land. He is buried in the military enclosure at Fort Douglas. (Hance, *Johnston, Connor, and The Mormons,* p. 145.)

[23]In the field near Fort Douglas.

Wiggins, Augustus W.	June '60-July '70	Contract Surgeon and Assistant Surgeon	Med Dept of George town College (Wash DC)
Williamson, Jonathan M.	Oct. '62-June '63, Nov. '63-March '64	Surgeon, California Volunteer	Unknown
Wilson, Alfred Davis	June '71	Assistant Surgeon	Univ Med Coll of NY
Wolcott, John G.	June '64-May '65, Oct. '65-Dec. '65[24]	Assistant Surgeon, New York Volunteer & Contract Surgeon	Unknown
Wolverton, William D.	Nov. '88-Oct. '91	Surgeon	Unknown
Wood, Marshall W.	Aug. '75-Oct. '75	Assistant Surgeon	Rush Med Coll (Chicago)

CAMP DUN GLEN

Davidsohn, Nathan	Jan '66-Feb '66	Contract Surgeon[25]	Unknown

FORT HALLECK

NAME	DATE/HALLECK	POSITION	EDUCATION
Azpell, Thomas F.	Aug. '71-Dec. '71	Assistant Surgeon	Jefferson Med Coll (Philadelphia)
Baldwin, William H.	Sept. '75-Nov. '75	Contract Surgeon	Jefferson Med Coll[26] (Philadelphia)
Brierly, Conant Bowdin[27]	Dec. '71-Apr. '72 July '72-Sept. '74	Contract Surgeon	Toland Med Coll (San Francisco)
Chismore, George			
	Sept. '72-Oct. '72	Contract Surgeon	Cooper Med Coll (San Francisco)[28]
Clark, Loren N.[29]	May '80-May '84 July '84-Dec. '85	Assistant Surgeon, First Lieutenant	Unknown
Corson, Edward Evan Watts	Aug. '74-Apr. '75	Contract Surgeon	Jefferson Med Coll (Philadelphia)
Dods, William B.[30]	July '71-Aug. '71	Contract Surgeon	Unknown

---

[24]After December 1865 Wolcott was stationed in Salt Lake City.

[25]Davidsohn's contract was annulled at Fort Churchill March 3, 1866, for refusing to face hostile Indians at Camp Dun Glen. National Archives, RG 94, E 561, B 147. Dun Glen was a small settlement of 250, mostly ranchers. Today the location is noted at an Interstate 80 intersection. The canyon, approximately 25 miles west of Winnemucca, had a temporary attachment of soldiers from Fort Churchill in the mid-1860s.

[26]*AMA Directory, 1918.*

[27]See Fort Churchill regarding Brierly's service.

[28]Harris, *California's Medical Story*, p. 139. The Medical College of the Pacific (reorganized as a Presbyterian College) became Cooper Medical College in 1882 and in 1912 became Stanford Medical School. After leaving Fort Halleck Chismore was in the class of 1873.

[29]See Fort McDermit regarding Clark's service.

[30]Dods was a member of the U.S. Colored Troops. See *Roster of Regimental Surgeons and Assistant Surgeons*, p. 239.

Dorr, Levi Lewis	July '71-Aug. '71	Contract Surgeon	Bellevue Hosp Med Coll (NYC)[31]
Harrison, John T.[32]	Sept. '69-Oct. '69	Contract Surgeon	Unknown
Haskins, Henry S.	Nov. '77-Apr. '79	Contract Surgeon	U of Mich[33]
Mckee, James Cooper	July '76	Surgeon, Major[34]	U of Pa (Philadelphia)
Newlands, William Sands	July '75-June '77	Assistant Surgeon, First Lieutenant	National Med Coll (Wash DC)
O'Reilly, Robert Maitland	Oct. '69-June '70	Assistant Surgeon, First Lieutenant	U of Pa (Philadelphia)[35]
Ord, James Lycurgus	June '79-Aug. '79	Contract Surgeon	Jefferson Med Coll (Philadelphia)[36]
Patty, Levi H.	May '70-July '71	Contract Surgeon	St. Louis Med Coll (St. Louis)
Polhemus, Adrian Suydam[37]	Dec. '85-Mar. '86 Apr. '86-Dec. '86	Assistant Surgeon	Bellevue Hosp Med Coll (NYC)
Pope, Benjamin Franklin	Nov. '68-Dec. '69	Assistant Surgeon, First Lieutenant[38]	Albany Med Coll (NY)
Rorke, James	Apr. '79-May '80	Contract Surgeon	U of Calif. (San Francisco)[39]
Semig, Bernard Gustavus[40]	Aug. '76-Sept. '76	Assistant Surgeon	U of Vienna (Austria)
Steele, Charles Harry	April '75-March '76	Contract Surgeon	U City of NY[41]
Steigers, Alonzo Francis[42]	March '83	Contract Surgeon	St. Louis Med Coll (St. Louis)
Stirling, Frank S.	July '67-Dec, '68	Contract Surgeon	Cooper Med Coll (San Francisco)[43]
Tallon, John E.	Sept. '77-Dec. '77	Contract Surgeon	U of Pa (Philadelphia)[44]
Tucker, Joseph E.	June '84-July '84	Contract Surgeon	U City of N Y[45]
West, Washington	May '72-July '72	Contract Surgeon	Washington U (St. Louis)[46]

[31]*AMA Directory, 1918* and *Medical Directory of the Pacific Coast.*

[32]See Forts Churchill and Ruby regarding Harrison's service.

[33]*California Medical Directory, 1878.* Also see McDermit regarding Haskins' service.

[34]Surgeon J. C. Mckee is noted in the hospital ledger on page 123 to be at Fort Halleck on June 25, 1876, but there is no indication of his position. National Archives, RG 112, E 88.

[35]National Archives, RG 112, E 88.

[36]*California Medical Directory.*

[37] See Forts McDermit and Scott regarding Polhemus' service.

[38]Pope was a volunteer during the Civil War but later was examined and received a commission.

[39]*Official Registry of Physicians and Surgeons in the State of California in 1885.*

[40]See Fort McDermit regarding Semig's service.

[41]Ibid.

[42]See Fort McDermit regarding Steigers' service.

[43]See footnote under Burns, at Fort Churchill.

[44]*Official Registry of Physicians and Surgeons in the State of California in 1885.*

[45]Ibid.

[46]*JAMA*, Volume L, Number 7, 1908, p. 555.

Woodhull, Alfred Alexander	June '77-Sept. '77	Surgeon, Major	U of Pa (Philadelphia)[47]

FORT HARNEY

NAME	DATE / HARNEY	POSITION	EDUCATION
Baker, William D.	Aug. '72-Sept. '73	Contract Surgeon	Unknown
Bartholf, John Henry	Nov. '74-Oct. '78	Assistant Surgeon	Coll Phy Surg, NY
Byrne, Charles B.	Sept. '69-July '71	Contract Surgeon & Assistant Surgeon	U of Pa[48] (Philadelphia)
Durrant, Henry	Sept. '73-Jan. '74	Contract Surgeon	NY Med Coll
Griffith, Edgar Milton	Aug. '78-Jan. '79	Contract Surgeon	Cooper Med Coll (San Francisco)
Hemenway, Stacy	June '76-Aug. '76	Contract Surgeon & Assistant Surgeon, Illinois Volunteer	Chicago Med Coll (NW Med Coll)
Knickerbocker, Bolivar	Nov. '73-Nov. '74	Assistant Surgeon	Jefferson Med Coll (Philadelphia)
Moffatt, Peter	Oct. '67-Sept. '69	Assistant Surgeon	Bellevue Hosp Med Coll (NYC)
Reynolds, Frank	July '71-Sept. '72	Assistant Surgeon	Royal Coll Surg of Dublin
Stirling, Frank S.	Oct. '78-June '80	Contract Surgeon	Cooper Med Coll

FORT INDEPENDENCE

NAME	DATE / INDEPENDENCE	POSITION	EDUCATION
Bentley, Edwin	April '76-May '76	Assistant Surgeon	Med Dept U of NY
Cronkhite, Henry M.	Dec '64-Oct. '66	Contract Surgeon	Albany Med Coll
Farnsworth, Amos	Oct. '67-April '68	Contract Surgeon	Unknown
Hoffman, David B.	Sept. '66-Dec '66	Contract Surgeon & Assistant Surgeon, California Volunteer	Unknown
Horn, George H.	July '62-Aug. '63	Assistant Surgeon & California Volunteer	Unknown
Keeney, Charles C.	Aug. '65-Sept. '65	Assistant Surgeon. Assigned to establish hospital	Jefferson Med Coll
Matthews, Washington	April '76-July '77	Assistant Surgeon	State U of Iowa Med Coll
McMillin, Thomas	Feb. '67-Aug. '70	Assistant Surgeon, Ohio Volunteer & Contract Surgeon	Unknown
Steele, Charles Harry	June '75-July '75	Contract Surgeon	U City of NY
White, Charles Braman	July '70-May '76	Assistant Surgeon	Med Dept U of La

---

[47] *AMA Directory, 1918.*

[48] *Directory of Deceased American Physicians,* p. 278.

FORT MCDERMIT

NAME	DATE /MCDERMIT	POSITION	EDUCATION
Axt, Godfrey H. T. Ferdinand	Aug. '67-Oct. '68	Contract & Assistant Surgeon (10/67)	U City of NY
Campbell, George	Nov. '72-Mar. '73	Contract Surgeon	Cooper Med Coll (San Francisco)[49]
Chapin, Samuel Farnum[50]	Aug. '65-Oct. '65	Contract Surgeon	U of Mich
Clark, Loren N.[51]	May '72-Aug. '72	Assistant Surgeon, First Lieutenant	Unknown
Corbusier, William Henry	July '69-Nov. '72	Assistant Surgeon, First Lieutenan	Bellevue Hosp Med Coll (NYC)
Gregory, John R.	Mar. '73-Oct. '73	Contract Surgeon	Coll Phys Surg (NYC)[52]
Griffith, Edgar Milton	June '78[53]	Contract Surgeon	Cooper Med Coll (San Francisco)
Gwyther, George[54]	Oct. '68-Aug. '69	Contract Surgeon	Unknown
Haskins, Henry S.[55]	May '73-Oct. '74	Contract Surgeon	U of Mich
Heinemann, John M.	June '78-July '78	Contract Surgeon	U of Calif (San Francisco)
Kendall, William Pratt	Sept. '85-Jan. '89	Assistant Surgeon	Columbia U Med Coll (NYC)
Kober, George Martin	Nov. '74-June '77	Contract Surgeon	Med Dept Georgetown Coll (Wash., D.C.)
Matthews, Washington	June '78	Assistant Surgeon[56]	State U of Iowa Med Coll
Polhemus, Adrian Suydam[57]	Sept. '84-Sept. '85	Assistant Surgeon	Bellevue Hosp Med Coll (NYC)
Semig, Bernard Gustavus[58]	July '77-Nov. '78	Assistant Surgeon	U of Vienna (Austria)
Smith, Andrew C.	June '78-July '78	Contract Surgeon	Cooper Med Coll (San Francisco)[59]
Snow, Thomas H.	Oct. '65-Jan. '67	Contract Surgeon	Cooper Med Coll (San Francisco)[60]

---

[49]*Directory of Deceased American Physicians,* p. 238.

[50]See Fort Churchill regarding Chapin's service.

[51]See Fort Halleck. regarding Clark's service.

[52]*Official Registry of Physicians and Surgeons in the State of California in 1885.*

[53]In field at Camp Willow Creek near Fort McDermit.

[54]Gwyther was a volunteer surgeon of the New Mexico 1st Cavalry during the Civil War. See *Roster of Regimental Surgeons and Assistant Surgeons,* p. 117. Also see Fort Ruby regarding Gwyther's service.

[55]See Fort Halleck regarding Haskins' service.

[56]Matthews was an assistant surgeon in the U. S. Veteran Volunteers during the Civil War. See *Roster of Regimental Surgeons and Assistant Surgeons,* pp. 253 and 254.

[57]See Forts Halleck and Scott regarding Polhemus' service.

[58]See Fort Halleck regarding Semig's service.

[59]*Official Registry of Physicians and Surgeons in the State of California in 1885.*

[60]*Registry of Physicians and Surgeons in California in 1887.*

Steigers, Alonzo Francis[61]	June '83-Oct. '84	Contract Surgeon	St. Louis Med Coll (St. Louis)
Todd, David Bryon	Oct. '78-June '83	Contract Surgeon	U of Mich[62]
Walker, Milton Monroe	Sept. '86-Nov. '86	Contract Surgeon	U of Md[63]

FORT MCGARRY

NAME	DATE/MCGARRY	POSITION	EDUCATION
Biggers, James W.[64]	Aug. '66-Mar. '67	Contract Surgeon	Unknown
Damour, Ferdinand	Nov. '67-Jan. '69	Contract Surgeon	U of Cal (San Francisco)[65]
Handy, John Charles	Feb. '67-Oct. '67	Contract Surgeon	No Diploma, studied with Dr. E. S. Cooper (San Francisco)[66]
Kisffy, Siegesmund	Feb. '66-Sept. '66	Contract Surgeon	U of Pesth[67] (Hungary)
Woods, Eugene H.	Oct. '65-Apr. '66	Contract Surgeon	Unknown

FORT NYE

NAME	DATE/NYE	POSITION	EDUCATION
Eversfield, William Octavus	Nov. '64-Nov. '65	Contract Surgeon	U of Pa (Philadelphia)
Munckton, George	Oct. '64-Dec. '64	Contract Surgeon	Unknown

FORT RAWLINS

NAME	DATE/RAWLINS	POSITION	EDUCATION
Wilson, Alfred Davis	Oct. '70-July '71	Assistant Surgeon	U Med Coll of NY (NYC)

FORT RUBY

NAME	DATE/RUBY	POSITION	EDUCATION
Biggers, James W.[68]	June '67-June '68	Contract Surgeon	Unknown
Brown, Isaac W.[69]	July '63-May '64	Assistant Surgeon, First Lieutenant, California Volunteer	Unknown

---

[61]See Fort Halleck regarding Steigers' service.

[62]*Registry of Physicians and Surgeons in California in 1887.*

[63]*AMA Directory, 1906.*

[64]See Fort Ruby regarding Biggers' service.

[65]*AMA Directory, 1906.*

[66]Although Handy (RG 94, 561) stated when he signed his contract that he had no diploma the *Medical Directory of the Pacific Coast,* lists him as a graduate from the Toland Medical College.

[67]See page 56 regarding Kisffy's credentials.

[68]See Fort McGarry regarding Biggers' service.

[69]Brown was a member of the 3rd Battalion Mountaineers, California Volunteers. See Fort Churchill regarding Brown's service.

Gwyther, George[70]	July '68-Oct. '68	Contract Surgeon	Unknown
Harrison, John T.[71]	Aug. '69-Sept. '69	Contract Surgeon	Unknown
Kinsman, John H.	May '68-Apr. '69	Assistant Surgeon	Harvard Med Coll
Kirke, Henry M.	Sept. '68-May '69	Assistant Surgeon	Jefferson Med Coll (Philadelphia)
Kirkpatrick, Charles A.	Sept. '62-Aug. '63	Assistant Surgeon	U of Cal (San Francisco)[72]
Long, John W.	May '64-June '67	Contract Surgeon	Bellevue Hosp Med Coll (NYC)[73]
Reid, Robert King	Sept. '62	Contract Surgeon and Surgeon[74]	Jefferson Med Coll & U of Pa (Philadelphia)
Williamson, Jonathan M.	Sept. '62	Surgeon, California Volunteer	Unknown

FORT SCOTT

NAME	DATE/SCOTT	POSITION	EDUCATION
Cassell, Francis M.[75]	Nov. '66-July '67	Contract Surgeon	Unknown
Denicke, Frederick	Oct. '69-Feb. '71	Contract Surgeon	No diploma, studied in Jena, Germany[76]
Dods, William B.	Oct. '69	Contract Surgeon	Unknown
Hayes, Lewis W.	June '67-May '68	Assistant Surgeon	Unknown
Spalding, Z. N.	June '65[77]	Contract Surgeon	Unknown
Watkins, John C.	May '68-Apr. '69	Contract Surgeon	Unknown

FORT THREE FORKS (WINTHROP)

NAME	DATE/THREE Forks	POSITION	EDUCATION
Cochrane, Adam H.	Sept. '66-Oct. '66	Contract Surgeon	Unknown

---

[70]See Fort McDermit regarding Gwyther's service.

[71]See Forts Churchill and Halleck regarding Harrison's service.

[72]Kirkpatrick was a volunteer assistant surgeon in the 3rd Battalion Mountaineers of California. See *Roster of Regimental Surgeons and Assistant Surgeons*, p. 2. See Charles A. Kirkpatrick Manuscript in the University of California Bancroft Library. In 1847 he attended lectures at the Ohio Medical College, and in 1871, after military service, graduated from the University of California. Also see "Medical School Directory of Graduates 1864-1921," *Univ. Cal. Bull.*, Third Series v. XV, no. 3,

[73]JAMA, Feb. 3, 1906, p. 375. There is a note in National Archives, RG 94, 561 of Long's file that Dr. Len Broeck kept no records of the accounts, but there is no further information on Broeck.

[74]Reid was a member of the 3rd Battalion Mountaineers of the California Volunteers.

[75]Cassell was assigned to Camp McKee, (Granite Creek, Nev.) on 20 June 1866 to relieve Assistant Surgeon William Grave Deal, a member of U.S. Colored Troops, 12th Infantry from Colfax, La. See *Roster of Regimental Surgeons and Assistant Surgeons*, p. 238. Deal was a member of the California Medical Society and a graduate of the Univ. of Maryland. See *Pacific Med. Surgi. J.*, v. 1, 1858, p. 497.

[76]When Denicke signed a contract with the army he wrote that he had no diploma, but the *Medical Directory of the Pacific Coast*, lists him as a graduate of the University of Göttengin, Germany.

[77]Spalding signed a contract in Susanville, August, 1864, and accompanied troops to Paradise Valley, May, 1865, later the site of Fort Scott, National Archives, RG 94, E 561, Box 541.

Colmache, Edward	April '66-June '71	Contract Surgeon	Unknown
Davis, W. H.	Sept. '70-Dec. '70	Unknown	Unknown

FORT WARNER

NAME	DATE/WARNER	POSITION	EDUCATION
Belt, Joseph C.	May '67-Aug. '67	Contract Surgeon	Unknown
Byrne, Charles B.	Aug. '71-July '73	Contract Surgeon & Assistant Surgeon	U of Pa (Philadelphia)
Cochrane, Adam H.	Oct. '66-April '67[78]	Contract Surgeon	Unknown
Colmache, Edward	Aug. '66-Sept. '66	Contract Surgeon	Unknown
Dickson, John M.[79]	Nov. '67-July '68	Assistant Surgeon	Unknown
Dods, William B.	Nov. '69	Contract Surgeon	Unknown
Dorr, Levi Lewis	Sept. '71- Mar '72	Contract Surgeon	Bellevue Hosp Med Coll (NYC)
Knight, Cyrus W.	April '71-Aug. '71	Contract Surgeon	Unknown
Nestell, Daniel D. T.	Oct. '69-June '70[80]	Contract Surgeon	Unknown
Phillips, Henry J.	July '73-Aug. '74	Assistant Surgeon, Captain	St Andrew, Scotland
Powell, Richard A.	Oct. '67-Oct. '69	Assistant Surgeon	Royal Coll Surg, Ireland
Tompkins, William A.	Sept. '67	Contract Surgeon	Unknown
Wiggins, Augustus W.	Dec. 69-May '70	Assistant Surgeon	Med Dept of Georgetown College (Wash DC)

---

[78]With the Wheeler Mapping Expedition in So. Calif. and Nev., April 1871 to Jan. 1872.

[79]Dickson was assigned to Fort Warner during Surgeon Powell's illness. He (Dixon/Dickson) is mentioned on various occasions by Gillis, *So Far From Home*, pp. 154, 158, and 177.

[80]With the Wheeler Mapping Expedition in So. Calif. and Nev., June to Oct. 1870.

Bryant's Letter about the Pyramid Lake War

Downieville, [California], May 31, 1860

My dear Father: Your letters of April 20th and May 5th have been received. The latter were received to-day. Most sincerely do Marie and myself thank you for your kind congratulations. In receiving the approbation of my parents we are rendered if possible more happy. We are both well and in enjoyment of reasonable prosperity. I was prevented from writing to you by the last mail by circumstances unavoidable. I left home for a visit to Utah to look after some of my debtors and some mining claims and barely got back with my scalp. I anticipated no danger when I left but the war commenced about the same time. I did not learn the news until I had arrived in the Indian country. I met trains of people and stock on their way to California, flying from the Indians. I made my way back but did not get time to write before I was obliged to return. How narrowly I escaped I have not time at present to detail. The Major (my father in law) was at Virginia City at the time. When I arrived in town news of the battle and defeat of the whites had reached here and the excitement was terrible. I found dispatches for me from the Major (as I was the only officer of his staff here) to have all of the arms & ammunition of the battalion conveyed immediately to the scene of action. I left on the following morning with an escort of 150 men—mostly volunteers under command of the sheriff of this county who was chosen to provide for the men until they arrived at Virginia City. Many who went lost friends or relatives in the battle. The arms were U.S. rifles or muskets. We arrived there after five days march. Our beds were the ground without shelter—one night of snow-storm and our food bacon and flour and water baked together. Ice every night. But all were healthy and hungry. The distance is 100 miles. We escaped from any attack. The details of the trip you will find in the Sierra Citizen. I found an Indian Boy (who had got frightened & run away the day before I got home) with his tribe on the Truckee river fishing. He told me that he wanted to come back—but was afraid someone would kill him because he was an Indian. His tribe (the Washoes) are friendly. The hostile Indians the Paiutes-Shoshones and Pitt river Indians number in all about 15,000 warriors well armed mostly with rifles from the Mormons and Hudson Bay Co. and abundant ammunition, a great deal of which has been thoughtlessly sold to them by our miners. About half of them are well mounted on fine horses. They were apparently friendly until about a month since when in a single night every Indian disappeared from the settlements and mining camps. They assembled at Pyramid Lake a few miles below Virginia City, held a council of war and determined to wipe out the whites. Then came daily news of massacres by the red villains. Ever since the discovery of these silver mines at Virginia City, they have complained and threatened that the neighborhood is their last and only resting place, California being on their west and east of them the great desert. On the 9th of this month a party of 105 men well mounted and well armed left Virginia City in search of parties of miners who were out prospecting and who were supposed to have been killed by the Indians. On the 12th they fell in with a large band of warriors near the pass where the Truckee river enters into Pyramid Lake. A hard and bloody battle was fought and the whites defeated. An expedition has now started after them under command of Col. Jack Hays and Major Hungerford—aided by a company of U. S. artillery and one of dragoons. I employed or rather found a man to represent me in the battalion as surgeon and after attending to the wounded returned to my business. Col. Hays was very anxious to have me remain but the Major and myself thought I had better be at home. Last night I received a dispatch that an attack was made upon the camp of the troops on the night of the 27th by 200 mounted Indians. 7 Indians killed and 3 of our men wounded. I expect while I am writing that a bloody bath is going on. The Major is now in his glory. Today is the one appointed for the attack upon Pyramid Lake. Hays, you will remember, was chief of the Texas rangers. The Major and him fought side by side in Mexico. The scene of the battleground where battle of the 12th was fought is horrible beyond description. The savages were not content with scalping their victims but after stripping them mutilated their bodies in a horrible manner. About 35 of the whites were killed and only about 15 Indians. I can give you further particulars in my next letter.

I acknowledge receipt of those receipts from Uncle Lank and yourself and send you a draft enclosed. Please pay $100 of it to Uncle Lank. I have written to him also by this mail to that office. The Indian war has killed business. It is a truly lamentable affair. The health of the town is excellent and my receipts clear of expense are at present not exceeding $5 per day in cash—and credit accounts are not reliable. It has never been so dull since I have been in the country. I will do as you have requested after this—that is to send the drafts by the last mail in each month. Your advice to me concerning money matters I can fully appreciate. Money and knowledge of my position which I [illegible] did by [illegible] to be able to shed occasionally a little sunshine upon the chill atmosphere which has so long surrounded our family. I look forward with great earnestness to the time when we shall meet again and knowing that it depends upon me to a certain extent. I am combining all of my powers of industry and economy to bring it about. The time is not far distant. Your views of spiritualism interested me. I have believed in earnest for three years, but I think that I have exercised good judgment in saying nothing about it. By speaking of it, I had nothing to gain and would subject myself to derision. I say I believe in it—I will qualify that by saying that it is more reasonable than any other theory concerning the destiny of man after this stage of existence. I have seen since I have been in Cal. suffice to satisfy me that all of these phenomena are not delusions. I often feel impulses come upon me suddenly as if given to me by some mysterious agency and at a moment when my mind would be employed with matters entirely foreign to the promptings of the impulse. I have performed surgical operations with the most perfect success that I did not feel as though I understood satisfactorily and yet after commencing the operation I would receive promptings in the same way as I was prompted to begin them, yet I dare not say to the world that I believe that a guardian spirit guides me. On this Indian expedition I passed through days that no one else would do by going by night to an Indian camp and I felt perfectly assured that all was safe. I was advised to take a certain road all of them being strange to me—yet my impulse was toward the road that I did take and if I had taken the other I would have been killed. There is a cause for all of this. I do not seek to know it because I believe it is not to be understood in this stage of existence. It would be of great detriment to the world at large if the nature of these things were known. Churches and mysterious ceremonies do much good in the world by controlling the ignorant and superstitious. Men of good minds should never make the subject of spiritualism an earnest topic of conversation except on rare occasions. For it avails nothing to themselves or others if they convert others to the belief. Let every man think for himself unless he makes it a business to think for others on matters of religion. Religious prejudice is impregnable. You must forbear the receipt of Marie's portrait for the present as it is impossible to get one without going to Marysville for it and that would cost over $100. During the summer there will be someone travelling through the place for the purpose of taking pictures. You shall have it by the first opportunity. Tell little Willie that he must excuse me for not consulting him before my marriage but next time I get married he shall know all about it before hand. When I come home I will bring him a piece of wedding cake. Tell mother that Marie has not in the least encroached upon her place in my heart. She is my angel mother still. Not a day passes but I think of her. Well, father, I expect you will think me a bore if I turn over the other page and will regard this letter as insipidly long as some of my others have been inexcusably short—so I will close by sending you my best love as well as Marie's who also writes to you by this mail. Her last letter was mislaid and did not get to the Post Office.

I am as ever your affectionate son

/s/ Edmund G. Bryant[1]

---

[1] A copy of this letter was given to Maggie Lowther, County Recorder and Auditor of Storey Co., Virginia City, Nev., by Betty Lowtrip. The original letter was found by her father at a NYC sidewalk sale of items from an apartment house that was to be demolished so that the Empire State Building could be built. The original letter is in her possession.

Fort Churchill Hospitalizations
July 1860 to January 1862[1]

Personnel Strength	280	284	283	182	210	209	205
Month/Year	7/60	8/60	9/60	10/60	11/60	12/60	1/61
Intermittent fever	6	8	5	5	3	11	9
Diarrhea	2	2	7	3	2	1	2
Rheumatism	5	3	3	5	6	4	5
Trauma	5	2	5	2	2	5	1
Catarrh	-	-	2	2	5	12	8
Tonsillitis	1	-	2	1	2	4	4
Ophthalmia	1	1	1	-	1	-	-
Digestive complaints	1	-	6	1	-	-	-
Constipation	-	-	1	1	1	-	-
Neuralgia	-	-	-	-	-	-	3
Syphilis	2	2	-	-	1	2	-
Gonorrhea	-	-	-	-	-	-	-
Bronchitis	-	-	-	2	1	2	-
Subcutaneous abscess	-	1	1	-	-	-	-
Paronychia	-	2	-	-	-	-	-
Delirium tremens	-	-	-	-	-	-	-
Hepatitis	-	-	-	-	-	-	-
Hemorrhoids	1	1	-	-	-	-	-
Pleuritis	-	-	-	-	1	2	-
Otitis	-	-	-	-	-	-	-
Toothache	-	-	-	-	-	-	1
Lumbago	1	-	-	1	-	-	1
Orchitis	1	-	-	-	-	-	-
Pneumonia	-	-	-	-	-	-	1
Scrofula	1	-	-	-	-	-	-
Scorbutus	-	-	-	-	-	-	-
Other	1	3	3	4	2	2	1
Total	28	25	36	27	27	45	36

Note: During this period there were three deaths; one from enteritis; one from typhoid; and one from intermittent fever. The few skin diseases are included under the heading of "other."

Fort Churchill Hospitalizations 2/61 to 8/61

| Personnel Strength | 207 | 198 | 193 | 209 | 297 | 204 | 199 |
Month/Year	2/61	3/61	4/61	5/61	6/61	7/61	8/61
Intermittent fever	4	9	8	7	3	7	6
Diarrhea	-	-	-	2	2	4	12
Rheumatism	3	4	5	3	1	4	7
Trauma	3	2	1	4	4	8	4
Catarrh	2	2	1	1	2	-	2
Tonsillitis	-	5	-	-	-	4	1
Ophthalmia	-	-	3	2	3	2	-
Digestive complaints	-	1	-	-	1	3	2
Constipation	-	-	-	-	-	2	2
Neuralgia	2	-	2	2	2	-	1
Syphilis	-	-	-	-	1	1	1
Gonorrhea	-	-	-	-	3	-	1
Bronchitis	-	-	-	1	-	-	2
Subcutaneous abscess	1	-	1	1	2	1	-
Paronychia	-	-	-	-	-	1	4
Delirium tremens	-	-	1	4	2	2	-
Hepatitis	-	-	-	-	-	-	5
Hemorrhoids	-	-	-	-	1	2	-
Pleuritis	-	-	-	-	1	-	
Otitis	-	-	-	1	1	-	-
Toothache	1	-	-	-	1	-	-
Lumbago	-	-	-	-	-	-	-
Orchitis	1	-	-	-	-	-	-
Pneumonia	-	-	-	-	-	-	-
Scrofula	-	-	-	-	-	-	-
Scorbutus	1	-	-	-	-	-	-
Other	5	-	1	2	6	2	3
Total	23	23	23	30	35	44	53

Fort Churchill Hospitalizations 9/61 to 1/62

Personnel Strength	207	198	193	209		
Month/Year	9/61	10/61	11/61	12/61		
					Total	%
Intermittent fever	8	10	2	10	121	18.3
Diarrhea	22	8	4	4	77	11.6
Rheumatism	5	6	1	2	72	10.9
Trauma	9	3	1	6	67	10.2
Catarrh	5	10	3	3	60	9.1
Tonsillitis	1	-	-	-	25	3.8
Ophthalmia	-	3	1	2	20	3.0
Digestive complaints	3	2	-	-	20	3.0
Constipation	1	5	2	4	19	2.9
Neuralgia	2	2	-	2	18	2.7
Syphilis	-	-	4	4	18	2.7
Gonorrhea	1	-	6	3	14	2.1
Bronchitis	1	1	-	3	13	2.0
Subcutaneous abscess	1	1	1	-	11	1.7
Paronychia	2	-	-	-	9	1.4
Delirium tremens	-	-	-	-	9	1.4
Hepatitis	2	-	-	1	8	1.2
Hemorrhoids	1	-	-	-	6	0.9
Pleuritis	1	-	-	-	5	0.8
Otitis	1	1	-	-	4	0.6
Toothache	1	-	-	-	4	0.6
Lumbago	-	-	-	-	3	0.5
Orchitis	-	-	1	-	3	0.5
Pneumonia	-	-	-	1	2	0.3
Scrofula	-	-	-	-	1	0.2
Scorbutus	-	-	-	-	1	0.2
Other	3	4	6	2	50	7.6
Total	70	56	32	47	660	100.0

Appendix V

Diagnoses of Patients
Admitted to Saint Mary Louise Hospital
March 1876 to November 1877

Month/Year	3/76	4/76	5/76	6/76	7/76	8/76	9/76
Typhoid/typhus	–	–	–	–	2	–	12
Trauma	–	–	2	4	1	4	3
Fevers	–	1	2	2	1	6	1
Subcutaneous abscess	–	–	–	1	–	1	2
Nervous debility	–	–	–	–	–	1	–
Consumption	–	1	–	–	1	1	3
Pneumonia	–	4	–	–	–	1	–
Rheumatism	–	–	–	1	2	–	–
Diarrhea	–	–	–	–	–	–	–
Erysipelas	–	–	–	1	–	–	1
Nervous sys disease	2	–	1	–	–	–	–
Salivated (syphilis)	–	–	–	–	–	–	–
Digestive complaints	–	–	–	1	–	–	3
Liver disease	–	–	–	–	–	–	1
Burns	1	–	–	–	–	2	–
Sore leg/finger/arm	–	–	–	–	–	–	–
Delirium tremens	–	–	–	–	–	–	3
Amputation	–	–	–	–	–	–	–
Ophthalmia	–	–	–	–	–	–	–
Insanity	–	–	–	–	–	–	–
Enlarged veins	–	–	–	–	–	–	–
Bronchitis	–	–	–	–	–	–	–
Pleuritis	–	–	–	–	–	–	1
Diphtheria	–	–	–	–	–	–	–
Cancer/throat	–	–	–	–	–	–	–
Asthma	–	–	–	–	–	–	–
Cramps	–	–	–	–	–	–	–
Dropsy	1	–	–	–	–	–	–
Anal fistula	–	–	1	–	–	–	–
Total	4	6	6	10	7	16	30

Diagnoses of Patients admitted to Saint Mary Louise Hospital
March 1876 to November 1877

Month/Year	10/76	11/76	12/76	1/77	2/77	3/77	4/77
Typhoid/typhus	12	6	2	–	1	1	1
Trauma	2	4	3	3	1	2	2
Fever	–	3	1	–	1	1	1
Subcutaneous abscess	1	4	1	4	–	3	2
Nervous debility	–	–	1	2	2	1	1
Consumption	2	1	–	–	–	2	2
Pneumonia	2	1	2	1	–	–	–
Rheumatism	–	–	2	–	–	1	1
Diarrhea	–	–	–	–	–	1	2
Erysipelas	2	2	–	–	–	1	–
Nervous sys disease	1	1	3	–	–	–	–
Salivated (syphilis)	–	–	–	–	–	1	2
Digestive complaints	1	–	–	–	–	–	–
Liver disease	–	–	–	–	1	–	–
Burns	–	–	–	–	–	–	–
Sore leg/finger/arm	–	1	–	1	1	–	–
Delirium tremens	–	–	–	–	–	–	–
Amputation	–	–	1	–	–	1	–
Ophthalmia	–	–	1	–	–	–	1
Insanity	–	–	–	–	–	–	1
Enlarged veins	–	–	–	–	–	1	–
Bronchitis	1	–	–	–	–	–	–
Pleuritis	–	–	–	–	–	–	–
Diphtheria	–	–	–	–	–	–	1
Cancer/throat	–	–	–	–	–	–	–
Asthma	–	–	–	–	–	–	1
Cramps	–	–	–	–	–	–	–
Dropsy	–	–	–	–	–	–	–
Anal fistula	–	–	–	–	–	–	–
Total	24	23	17	11	7	16	18

Diagnoses of Patients admitted to Saint Mary Louise Hospital March 1876 to November 1877

Month/Year	5/77	6/77	7/77	8/77	9/77	10/77	Total	%
Typhoid/typhus	2	1	2	1	9	2	54	18.2
Trauma	2	3	4	4	5	2	51	17.2
Fevers (all)	–	–	3	2	5	1	31	10.4
Abscess/inflame	1	1	–	1	1	–	23	7.7
Nervous debility	2	2	1	2	3	4	22	7.4
Consumption	–	–	1	2	1	1	18	6.1
Pneumonia	2	–	–	–	1	–	14	4.7
Rheumatism	1	–	–	1	–	4	13	4.4
Diarrhea	–	3	3	–	–	1	10	3.4
Erysipelas	–	–	–	1	–	–	8	2.7
Nervous sys disease	–	–	–	–	–	–	8	2.7
Salivated (syphilis)	–	–	4	1	–	–	8	2.7
Digestive complaints	–	–	–	–	–	–	5	1.7
Liver disease	1	–	–	–	1	–	4	1.3
Burns	–	–	–	–	1	–	4	1.3
Sore leg/finger/arm	–	–	–	–	1	–	4	1.3
Delirium tremens	–	–	–	–	–	–	3	1.0
Amputation	–	–	–	1	–	–	3	1.0
Ophthalmia	–	–	–	1	–	–	3	1.0
Insanity	–	1	–	–	–	–	2	1.0
Enlarged veins	–	–	–	–	–	–	1	0.7
Bronchitis	–	–	–	–	–	–	1	0.7
Pleuritis	–	–	–	–	–	–	1	0.7
Diphtheria	–	–	–	–	–	–	1	0.7
Cancer/throat	–	1	–	–	–	–	1	0.7
Asthma	–	–	–	–	–	–	1	0.7
Cramps	–	–	–	1	–	–	1	0.7
Dropsy	–	–	–	–	–	–	1	0.7
Anal fistula	–	–	–	–	–	–	1	0.7
Total	11	12	18	18	28	15	297	100%

Bibliography

BOOKS

Ackerknecht, Erwin H. *Malaria in the Upper Mississippi Valley 1760-1900*. Balto: Johns Hopkins Univ. Press, 1945.

Adams, George Worthington. *Doctors in Blue: The Medical History of the Union Army in the Civil War*. NY: Henry Schuman, 1952.

Addenbrooke, Alice Baltzelle. *The Enchanted Fort*. Sparks, Nevada: Western Printing & Pub. Co., 1968.

Adjutant General's Office. *Orders and Special Orders, Department of California, 1860*.

American Medical Association Directory, 1906. Chicago: AMA, 1906.

American Medical Association Directory, 1918. Chicago: AMA, 1918.

Angel, Myron, ed. *History of Nevada with Illustrations and Biographical Sketches of its Prominent Men and Pioneers*. Oakland: Thompson and West, 1881. Reissued, Berkeley: Howell-North, 1958. Poulson, Helen J. *Index to Thompson and West's History of Nevada*, Bibliographical Series, no. 6. Carson City: Univ. Nev. Press, 1966.

Annual Reports of the Surgeon General of the Army. Washington: SGO, 1860-1869, 1871-1874, 1876-1889.

Armstrong, Robert D., *A Preliminary Union Catalog of Nevada Manuscripts*. Reno: Univ. of Nev. Library, 1967.

Ashburn, Percy M., *A History of the Medical Department of the United States Army*. Boston: Houghton Mifflin Co., 1929.

Barry, Patricia A., *In Search of Captain Warner*. Bend, Oregon: Maverick Pub., 1995.

Bayne-Jones, Stanhope, *The Evolution of Preventive Medicine in the United States Army, 1607-1939*. Washington, D. C: SGO, 1968.

Beckham, Stephen Dow, *Land of the Umpqua: A History of Douglas County, Oregon*. Roseburg, Oregon: Douglas County Commissioners, 1986.

Berlin, Ellin, *Silver Platter*. Garden City, NY: Doubleday & Co. 1957.

Biddle, Ellen McGowan, *Reminiscences of a Soldier's Wife*. Philadelphia: J. B. Lippincott Co., 1907.

Biennial Report of the Adjutant General of the State of Nevada for the Years 1883 and 1884. Carson City, Nevada: John Church, State Printer, 1865.

Bowers, Nathan A., *Cone-Bearing Trees of the Pacific Coast.* Palo Alto: Pacific Books, 1961.

Boyd, Orsemus Bronson, Mrs. [Frances Anne Mullen Boyd], *Cavalry Life in Tent and Field.* NY: J. Selwin Tait & Sons, 1894 Lincoln: Univ. Nebr. Press, 1982.

Brown, Harvey E., *The Medical Department of the United States Army from 1775 to 1873.* Wash., D. C: SGO, 1873.

Burton, Richard R., *The City of the Saints, and Across the Rocky Mountains to California.* NY: Harper & Brothers, 1862.

Bush, Lester E. Jr., *Health and Medicine among the Latter-day Saints: Science, Sense, and Scripture.* NY: Crossroad Pub. Co., 1993.

Butler, Samuel W., *The Medical Register and Directory of the United States.* Philadelphia: Office of Medical & Surgical Reporter, 1877.

Bynum, W.F. and V. Nutton, eds., *Theories of Fever from Antiquity to the Enlightenment.* London: Wellcome Inst. Hist. Med., 1981.

California Medical Directory, 1878.

Catton, Bruce. *The Coming Fury.* Garden City, NY: Doubleday & Co., Inc., 1961.

Chapman, Arthur, *The Pony Express.* NY: A. L. Burt Co., 1932.

Chapman, Charleton B., *Order Out of Chaos: John Shaw Billings and America's Coming of Age.* Boston: Francis A. Countway Library of Medicine, 1994.

Circular No. 1. Report on Epidemic Cholera and Yellow Fever in the Army of the United States, During the Year 1867. Washington: GPO, 1868.

Circular No. 4. A Report on Barracks and Hospitals with Descriptions of Military Posts. Billings, J. S., Washington: GPO, 1870.

Circular No. 5. Report on Epidemic Cholera in the Army of the United States, During the Year 1866. Washington: GPO, 1867.

Circular No. 8. A Report on the Hygiene of the United States Army with Descriptions of Military Posts. Washington: GPO, 1875.

Circular No. 9. A Report to the Surgeon General on the Transport of the Sick and Wounded by Pack Animals. Washington: 1877.

Circular No. 10. Approved Plans and Specifications for Post Hospitals. Washington: SGO, 1877.

Coffman, Edward M., *The Old Army: A Portrait of the American Army in Peace Time, 1784-1898.* NY: Oxford Univ. Press, 1986.

Coolidge, Richard, *Statistical Report on the Sickness and Mortality in the Army of the United States, ...Jan. 1839 to Jan.1855.* Washington, D. C: GPO, 1856.

Coolidge, Richard, *Statistical Report on the Sickness and Mortality in the Army of the United States, Compiled from the Records of the Surgeon General's Office, Embracing a period of Five Years, from Jan. 1855 to Jan. 1860.* Wash. D.C: GPO, 1860.

Corbusier, William T., *Verde to San Carlos: Recollections of a Famous Army Surgeon and His Observant Family on the Western Frontier, 1869-1886.* Tucson: Dale Stuart King, 1969.

Cosulich, Bernice, *Tucson.* Tucson: Arizona Silhouettes, 1953.

Cragen, Dorothy Clora, *The Boys in the Sky-Blue Pants: The Men and Events at Camp Independence and Forts of Eastern California, Nevada and Utah, 1862-1877.* Fresno: Pioneer Pub. Co., 1975.

Cunningham, H. H., *Doctors in Gray: The Confederate Medical Service.* Baton Rouge: La. State Univ. Press, 1958.

Dammann, Dr. Gordon, *Pictorial Encyclopedia of Civil War Medical Instruments and Equipment, Volume II.* Missoula, MT: Pictorial Histories Pub. Co., 1988.

Davis, Sam P., ed., *The History of Nevada,* 2 vols. Reno: Elms Pub. Co., 1913.

Davis, William Newell, Jr., *Sagebrush Corner: The Opening of California's Northeast.* NY: Garland Pub., 1974.

Directory of Deceased American Physicians 1804-1929. Chicago: AMA, 1993.

Doten, Alfred, Journals of, 1849-1903, 3 vols., Walter Van Tilburg Clark, ed., Reno: Univ. Nev. Press, 1973.

Drake, Daniel, *A Systematic Treatise, Historical, Etiological, and Practical on the Principal Diseases of the Interior Valley of North America, as They Appear in the ...,* 2 vols. Cincinnati: Winthrop B. Smith & Co., 1850.

Duffy, John, *The Healers: The Rise of the Medical Establishment.* NY: McGraw-Hill, 1976.

Dunlop, Richard, *Doctors of the American Frontier: A Tribute to the Healing Instinct of the Early American Medicine Men - and to the Stamina of their Patients.* Garden City, NY: Doubleday & Co., 1965.

Dunn, Jacob Piatt, *Massacres of the Mountains; A History of the Indian Wars of the Far West 1815-1875.* NY: Archer House, 1886.

Eben, R. J., Randy Emm, and Dorothy Nez, *Numa: A Northern Paiute History.* Reno: Inter-tribal Council Nev., 1976.

Egan, Ferol, *Sand in a Whirlwind: The Paiute Indian War of 1860.* Reno: Univ. Nev. Press, 1985.

Eggerth, Arnold H., *The History of the Hoagland Laboratory.* Brooklyn: 1960.

Elliott, Russell R., *History of Nevada.* Lincoln: Univ. Nebr. Press, 1973.

Flexner, Abraham, *Medical Education in the United States and Canada: A Report to the Carneigie Foundation for the Advancement of Teaching.* NY: 1910.

Frazer, Robert Walter, ed., *Mansfield on the Condition of the Western Forts, 1853-54.* Norman: Univ. Okla. Press, 1963.

Frazer, Robert Walter, *Forts of the West: Military Forts and Presidios and Posts Commonly Called Forts West of the Mississippi River to 1898.* Norman: Univ. Okla. Press, 1965.

Garnier, Pierre, *A Medical Journey in California,* Trans by L. Jay Oliva, Intro. and annotated by Doyce B. Nunis, Jr. Los Angeles: Zeitlin & Ver Brugge, 1967.

Garrison, Lieut. Col. Fielding H., *Notes on the History of Military Medicine.* Wash: Assn. of Milit. Surg., 1922.

Geiger, Vincent, and Wakeman Bryarly, *Trail to California: The Overland Journal of Vincent Geiger and Wakeman Bryarly,* Intro., by David Morris Potter. New Haven: Yale Univ. Press, 1945.

Gilbert, Frank T., *History of San Joaquin County.* Oakland, California: Thompson & West, 1879.

Gillett, Mary C., *The Army Medical Department, 1775-1818.* Washington, D. C: Center of Military History, 1981.

_____. *The Army Medical Department, 1818-1865.* Washington, D. C: Center of Military History, 1987.

Gilliss, Julia, *So Far from Home: An Army Bride on the Western Frontier, 1865-1869.* Portland: Oreg. Hist. Soc. Press, 1993.

Goetzmann, William H., *Army Exploration in the American West, 1803-1863.* New Haven: Yale Univ. Press, 1959.

Gould, Benjamin Apthorp, *Investigation in the Military and Anthropological Statistics of American Soldiers.* NY: Arno Press, 1979.

Haller, John S., Jr., *Medical Protestants: The Eclectics in American Medicine, 1825-1939.* Carbondale, IL: So. Ill. Univ. Press, 1994.

Hamilton, Frank Hastings, *A Treatise on Military Surgery and Hygiene.* NY: Bailliére Bros., 1865.

Hance, Irma Watson and Irene Warr, compilers by, *Johnston, Connor, and The Mormons: An Outline of Military History in Northern Utah.* Published in Commemoration of the 100th Anniversary of Fort Douglas, Utah, Oct. 22, 1962.

Handbook of North American Indian, V. 11, Great Basin. Wash: Smithsonian Inst., 1986.

Hardesty, Donald L., ed., *Historical, Architectural, and Archaeological Studies of Fort Churchill, Nevada.* Carson City, Nevada: Division of State Parks, 1978.

Harris, Henry, *California's Medical Story.* San Francisco: Grabborn Press, 1932.

Hart, Herbert M., *Old Forts of the Far West.* Seattle: Superior Pub. Co., 1965.

_____. *Old Forts of the Northwest.* NY: Bonanza Books, 1963.

_____. *Tour Guide to Old Western Forts.* Boulder: Pruett Pub. Co., 1980.

Hein, Lieutenant Colonel O[tto] L[ouis], *Memories of Long Ago: Prominent Persons Encountered and Noticeable Incidents Recalled, Before and During the Civil War, 1855-65; while Stationed on the Western Frontier, in the Early Seventies and Eighties; ...*NY: G. P. Putnam's Sons, 1925.

Heitman, Francis B. *Historical Register and Dictionary of the United States Army, From its Organization, December 29, 1789, to March 2, 1903, 2* vols. Washington: GPO, 1903.

Henderson, Thomas, *Hints on the Medical Examination of Recruits for the Army, and on the Discharge of Soldiers from the Service on Surgeon's Certificate.* Philadelphia: 1840.

Henley, Brigadier General David C., *Brigadier General Sylvester Churchill: The Story of an American Army Hero, together with the Saga of Nevada's Pioneer Fort Churchill and the Fighting Warship USS Churchill County.* Fallon, NV, West. Milit. Hist. Assn., 1988.

Henry, Guy V., *Military Record of Civilian Appointments in the United States Army, V. I.* NY: Carleton, 1869.

Henry, Robert S., *The Armed Forces Institute of Pathology: Its First Century 1862-1962.* Washington, D. C: SGO, 1964.

Hodges, Robert Edgar, "Vitamin C." Roslyn B. Alfin-Slater and David Kritchevsky eds., *Nutrition and the Adult: Micronutrients.* NY: Plenum Press, 1980.

Holloway, Lisabeth M., *Medical Obituaries: American Physicians' Biographical Notices in Selected Medical Journals Before 1907.* NY: Garland Pub., 1981.

Hume, Edgar Erskine, *Ornithologists of the United States Army Medical Corps: Thirty-Six Biographies.* Balto: Johns Hopkins Univ. Press, 1942.

Hume, Edgar Erskine, *Victories of Army Medicine: Scientific Accomplishments of the Medical Department of the United States Army.* Philadelphia: J. B. Lippincott Co., 1943.

Hunt, Aurora, *The Army of the Pacific, 1860-1866*. Glendale, California: Arthur H. Clark Co., 1951.

Hutton, Paul A., *Soldiers West: Biographies from the Military Frontier*. Lincoln: Univ. Nebr. Press, 1987.

Jocelyn, Stephen Perry, *Mostly Alkali*. Caldwell, Idaho: Caxton Printers, 1953.

Jones, J. Roy, *Memories, Men and Medicine: A History of Medicine in Sacramento, California*. Sacramento: Premier Pub., 1950.

Karolevitz, Robert F., *Doctors of the Old West, A Pictorial History of Medicine on the Frontier*. Seattle: Superior Pub. Co., 1967.

Kelly, Howard Atwood & Walter L. Burrage, *Dictionary of American Medical Biography*. NY: D. Appleton & Co., 1928.

Kelly, J. Wells, *Second Directory of Nevada Territory; etc.* Virginia, Nevada: 1863.

Keyes, Edward L., *The Surgical Diseases of the Genito-Urinary Organs including Syphilis*. NY: D. Appleton & Co., 1874.

_____. *Syphilis: A Treatise for Practitioners*. NY: D. Appleton & Co., 1908.

Kimball, Maria Brace, *A Soldier-Doctor of our Army: James P. Kimball, Late Colonel and Assistant Surgeon-General, U.S. Army*. Boston: Houghton Mifflin Co., 1917.

Knight, Oliver, *Life and Manner in the Frontier Army*. Norman: Univ. Okla. Press, 1978.

Kober, George Martin, *Reminiscences of George Martin Kober, M.D., LL.D.* Menasha, Wisconsin: George Banta Pub. Co., 1930.

Langley, Harold D., ed., *To Utah With the Dragoons and Glimpses of Life in Arizona and California 1858-1859*. Salt Lake City: Univ. Utah Press, 1974.

Laufe, Abe, ed. *An Army Doctor's Wife on the Frontier: Letters from Alaska and the Far West, 1874-1878*. Pittsburgh: Univ. Pittsburgh Press, 1962.

Lender, Mark Edward, and James Kirby Martin, *Drinking in America: A History*. NY: Free Press, 1982.

Lewis, Marvin, *Martha and the Doctor: A Frontier Family in Central Nevada*. Reno: Univ. Nev. Press, 1977.

Lewis, Oscar, *Silver Kings: The Lives and Times of Mackay, Fair, Flood, and O'Brien, Lords of the Nevada Comstock Lode*. NY: Alfred A. Knopf, 1947.

_____. *The War and the Far West: 1861-1865*. Garden City, NY: Doubleday, 1961.

Longstreth, Morris, *Rheumatism, Gout, and Some Allied Disorders.* NY; William Wood & Co., 1882.

Mack, Effie Mona, *History of Nevada.* Glendale, California: Arthur H. Clark Co., 1935.

————. *Mark Twain in Nevada.* NY: Charles Scribner's Sons, 1947.

Mathias, Peter, "Swords and Ploughshares: The Armed Forces, Medicine and Public Health in the late eighteenth Century," *War and Economic Development*, J. M. Winter, ed. Cambridge: Cambridge Univ. Press, 1975.

Mattes, Merrill J., *Indians, Infants and Infantry: Andrew and Elizabeth Burt on the Frontier.* Lincoln: Univ. Nebr. Press, 1960.

McKenneys' Gazetteer and Directory of the Central Pacific Railroad for 1871. Sacramento, CA: 1871.

McKenney's Pacific Coast Directory 1886-1887. San Francisco: L. M. McKenney & Co., 1886.

Medical Soc. State of Calif., 1891, v. 21. San Francisco: 1891.

Mercantile Guide and Directory for Virginia City, Gold Hill, Silver City and American City, etc. by Charles Collins. Virginia, Nevada: 1864-5.

Michelson, Miriam, *The Wonderlode of Silver and Gold.* Boston: Stratford Co., 1934.

Moorman, Donald R., and Gene A. Sessions, *Camp Floyd and the Mormons: The Utah War.* Salt Lake City: Univ. Utah Press, 1992)

National Union Catalogue of Manuscripts. Wash., D. C: Lib. Congress, 1959-90.

Nevada Directory, for 1868-69. by William Gillis Virginia, Nevada: 1868.

Norwood, William Frederick, *Medical Education in the United States Before the Civil War.* NY: Arno Press & New York Times, 1971.

Notson, William M., *Fort Concho Medical History, Jan.1869 to July 1872.* San Angelo, Texas: Fort Concho Preservation & Museum, 1974.

Numbers, Ronald L., ed., *The Education of American Physicians.* Berkeley: Univ. Calif. Press, 1980.

Oakes, Stanley C. Jr., et al , ed., *Malaria: Obstacles and Opportunities.* Washington, D.C: National Academy Press, 1991.

Official Register of Physicians and Surgeons in the State of California, 1885. San Francisco: Board of Examiners, 1885.

Official Register of Physicians and Surgeons in the State of California, 1887. San Francisco: Board of Examiners, 1887.

O'Malley, C. D., ed., *The History of Medical Education.* Berkeley: Univ. Cal. Press, 1970.

Orton, Richard H., *Records of California Men in the War of the Rebellion, 1861 to 1867*. Sacramento: State Office, 1890.

Pacific Coast Directory for 1871-72. by Henry G. Langley. San Francisco: 1871.

Pacific Coast Directory for 1880-1881. San Francisco: 1880.

Pacific Coast Directory for 1867: etc. by Langley 1867.

Pacific Medical and Surgical Journal, 1858-1890.

Paden, Irene D., *The Wake of the Prairie Schooner*. NY: Macmillan Co., 1943.

Paher, Stanley W., *Nevada Ghost Towns and Mining Camps*. Berkeley: Howell-North Books, 1970.

Paher, Stanley W., ed., research by Kathryn Totton, *Fort Churchill: Nevada Military Outpost of the 1860's*. Las Vegas: Nev. Pub., 1981.

Parker, James, *The Old Army: Memories, 1872-1918*. Philadelphia: Dorrance & Co., 1929.

Parkes, Edmund A., *A Manual of Practical Hygiene, With an Appendix giving the American Practice in Matters Relating to Hygiene*, ed. F. S. B. François de Chaumont 2 vols., NY: William Wood & Co., 1883.

Patterson, Edna B., *Sagebrush Doctors and Health Conditions of Northeast Nevada from Aboriginal Times to 1972*. Springville: Utah Art City Pub. Co., 1972.

Paul, Rodman Wilson, *Mining Frontiers of the Far West 1848-1880*. NY: Holt, Rinehart & Winston, 1963.

Phalen, James M., compiler, *Chiefs of the Medical Department United States Army 1775-1940*. Wash., D. C: Army Med. Lib., 1940.

Pilcher, James Evelyn, *The Surgeon Generals of the Army of the United States of America*. Carlisle, Pennsylvania: Assn. Military Surgeons, 1905.

Prucha, Francis Paul, *Broadax and Bayonet: The Role of the United States Army in the Development of the Northwest 1815-1860*. Madison, Wisconsin: State Hist. Soc., 1953.

_____. *A Guide to the Military Posts of the United States 1789-1895*. Madison, Wisconsin: State Hist. Soc., 1964.

Read, Jay Marion and Mary E. Mathes, *History of the San Francisco Medical Society*, V. 1, 1850-1900. San Francisco: James H. Barry, 1958.

Regulations for the Army of the United States. 1889. Washington: GPO, 1889.

Richards, Ralph T., *Of Medicine, Hospitals, and Doctors*. Salt Lake City: Univ. Utah Press, 1953.

Richmond, Phyllis Allen, "American Attitudes Toward the Germ Theory of Disease 1860-1880)," *Theory and Practice in American Medicine.* Gert H. Brieger, ed., NY: Sci. Hist. Pub., 1976.

Roberts, Robert B., *Encyclopedia of Historic Forts: The Military, Pioneer, and Trading Posts of the United States.* NY: Macmillan, 1988.

Rogers, Frederick Blackburn, *Fort Bidwell.* San Francisco: California, Dept. of Natural Resources, Div. of Beaches & Parks, May 19, 1959.

_____. *Soldiers of the Overland: Being Some Account of the Services of General Patrick Edward Connor and his Volunteers in the Old West.* San Francisco: Grabhorn Press, 1938.

Rorabaugh, W. J., *The Alcoholic Republic: An American Tradition.* NY: Oxford Univ. Press, 1979.

Rosen, George, *A History of Public Health.* NY: MD Pub., 1958.

_____. *The Structure of American Medical Practice 1874-1941.* Charles E. Rosenberg, ed., Philadelphia: Univ. of Penn. Press, 1983.

Rosenberg, Charles E., *The Cholera Years: The United States in 1832, 1849, and 1866.* Chicago: Univ. Chicago Press, 1962.

_____. *Explaining Epidemics and Other Studies.* NY: Cambridge Univ. Press, 1992.

Rothstein, William G., *American Physicians in the 19th Century: From Sects to Science.* Balto: Johns Hopkins Univ. Press, 1972.

Roster of Regimental Surgeons and Assistant Surgeons in the U.S. Army Medical Department During the Civil War. Gaithersburg, Maryland: Olde Soldier Books, 1989.

Russell, Paul F., *Man's Mastery of Malaria.* London: Oxford Univ. Press, 1955.

San Francisco Business Directory and Mercantile Guide for 1864-5. by B.F. Stilwell & Co. San Francisco: 1864.

Scrugham, James G., ed., *Nevada: A Narrative of the Conquest of a Frontier Land,* 3 v. Chicago: Amer. Hist. Soc., 1935.

Seagraves, Anne, *Women of the Sierra.* Lakeport, California: Wesanne Enterprises, 1990.

Senn, Nicholas, *Medico-Surgical Aspects of the Spanish American War.* Chicago, AMA Press, 1900.

Shryock, Richard H., *Medical Licensing in America, 1650-1965.* Balto: Johns Hopkins Univ. Press, 1967.

Simpson, Captain J. H., *Report of Explorations across the Great Basin of the Territory of Utah for a Direct Wagon-Route from Camp Floyd to Genoa, in Carson Valley, in 1859.* Wash: GPO, 1876.

Starr, Paul, *The Social Transformation of American Medicine.* NY: Basic Books, 1982.

Stewart, George R., *The California Trail: An Epic with Many Heroes.* Lincoln: Univ. Nebr. Press, 1962.

Stone, Eric, *Medicine Among the American Indians.* NY: 1932.

Storey, Ormsby, Washoe and Lyon Counties Directory for 1871-72. Sacramento: 1871.

Strümpell, Adolf, *Text-Book of Medicine,* NY: D. Appleton & Co., 1894.

Summerhayes, Martha, *Vanished Arizona: Recollections of the Army Life of a New England Woman.* Salem, Mass: Salem Press Co., 1911 Lincoln: Univ. Nebr. Press, 1979.

Temkin, Owsei, *The Double Face of Janus and Other Essays in the History of Medicine.* Balto: Johns Hopkins Univ. Press, 1977.

Thacher, James, *A Military Journal: 1775-1783.* Plymouth, Massachussetts, 1823.

Tondorf, Francis A., *Anniversary Tribute to George Martin Kober, in Celebration of his Seventieth Birthday by his Friends and Associates, March 28. 1920.* Washington, D.C: 1920.

Train, Percy, James R Henrichs and W. Andrew Archer, *Medicinal Uses of Plants by Indian Tribes of Nevada.* Lawrence, Massachussetts: Quarterman Pub., repr. rev. 1957 ed.

Tyler, Robert Ogden, *Revised Outlines and Descriptions of Posts and Stations of Troops in the Military Division of the Pacific.* San Francisco: Headquarters, 1872.

Tyson, James L., *Diary of a Physician in California.* Oakland, California: Bilbooks, 1955.

United States Army Regulations, of 1861, Revised. Washington: G.P.O., 1863.

Unruh, John D., *The Plains Across: The Overland Emigrants and the Trans-Mississippi West, 1840-60.* Chicago: Univ. of Ill. Press, 1982.

Utley, Robert Marshall, *Frontier Regulars: The United States Army and the Indian, 1866-1891.* NY: Macmillan Pub. Co., 1973.

Varley, James F., *Brigham and the Brigadier: General Patrick Connor and His California Volunteers in Utah and Along the Overland Trail.* Tucson: Westernlore Press, 1989.

Walker, M. R. [Morris Rollins], *Story of the Nevada State Society and Nevada Medicine.* 1937.

Walsham, William Johnson, *Surgery its Theory and Practice.* Philadelphia: P. Blakiston, Son & Co., 1887.

The War of the Rebellion: A Compilation of the Official Records of the Union and Confederate Armies. Series I–V. L, Part I–Reports, Correspondence, etc., Part II–Correspondence, etc. Washington: GPO, 1897.

Warner, John Harley, *The Therapeutic Prospective: Medical Practice, Knowledge, and Identity in America, 1820-1885.* Cambridge: Harvard Univ. Press, 1986.

Warshaw, Leon J., *Malaria: The Biography of a Killer.* NY: Rinehart & Co., 1949.

Whiting, J. S. and Richard J., *Forts of the State of California.* Longview, Washington: Daily News Press, 1960.

Wren, Thomas, *A History of the State of Nevada its Resources and People.* Chicago: Lewis Pub. Co., 1904.

Young, James Harvey, *The Toadstool Millionaires: A Social History of Patent Medicines in America before Federal Regulation.* Princeton: Princeton Univ. Press, 1961.

ARTICLES

Alexander, Thomas G. and Leonard J. Arrington, "The Utah Military Frontier, 1872-1912, Forts Cameron, Thornburgh, and Duchesne," *Utah Hist. Quart.* Fall 1964, pp. 330-354.

Baker, Samuel L., "Physician Licensure Laws in the United States, 1865-1915," *J. Hist. Med. & Allied Sci.,* 39 (1984) pp. 173-197.

Beckham, Stephen Dow, "Lonely Outpost: The Army's Fort Umpqua," *Oreg. Hist. Quart.,* Sept. 1969, pp. 233-254.

Bill, Joseph Howard, "Notes on Arrow Wounds," *Amer. J. Med. Sci.* (Oct., 1862) pp. 365-87.

Borden, Daniel L., "William Cline Borden 1858-1934," *Med. Ann. Dist. Columbia,* V, Sept. and Oct., 1936.

Breeden, James O., "Medicine in the West—An Introduction," *J. West,* XXI, no. 3 (July 1982) pp. 3-4.

Brieger, Gert H., "American Surgery and the Germ Theory of Disease," *Bull. Hist. Med.,* 40 (1966) pp. 135-45.

Brieger, Gert H., "Health and Disease on the Western Frontier—A Bicentennial Appreciation (Medicine in American History)," *West. J. Med.,* 125 (July 1976), pp. 28-35.

_____. "Medical Education in the Far West," *J. West,* XXI, no. 3 (July 1982), pp. 42-48.

Brimlow, George F., "The Life of Sarah Winnemucca: the Formative Years," *Oreg. Hist. Quart.,* v., LIII (June 1952), pp. 103-34.

Brody, Stuart A., "Hospitalization of the Mentally Ill During California's Early Years: 1849-1853," *Psy. Quart. Supplement*, Part 2 (1964).

Buckland, Samuel S., "Indian Fighting in Nevada," *Nev. Hist. Soc. Papers*, I, 1917, pp. 171-4.

Busey, Samuel C., "The Organization, High *Espirit De Corps*, High Standard of Education and Scientific Attainments of the Army Medical Department," *Address at the Closing Exercises of the Army Medical School, March 12, 1897, Washington, D. C.*, Washington, D. C: Gibson Bros., 1897.

Camargo, Carlos A., "1492—The Medical Consequences," *West. J. Med.*, 160, no. 6., June 1994, pp. 545-553.

Cammack, Sister Alberta, "A Faithful Account of the Life and Death of Doctor John Charles Handy," *Smoke Signal*, (Westerners, Tucson, 1989), no. 52, pp. 36-39.

Caum, Norman C., "Fort Douglas, Utah," *Recruiting News*, Dec, 1, 1923, pp. 6-7.

Clary, David A., "The Role of the Army Surgeon in the West: Daniel Weisel at Fort Davis, Texas, 1868-1872," *West. Hist. Quart*, III, (Jan. 1972), pp. 53-66.

Cline, I. M., "The Climatic Causation of Disease with Chart Showing the Pathological Distribution of Climate in the United States," *Proceed. Tex. State Med. Assn. 1895*.

Courtwright, David, "Opiate Addiction in the American West, 1850-1920," *J. West*, XXI, no. 3, (July 1982), pp. 23-31.

Cozen, Lewis N., "Military Orthopedic Surgery," *Clin. Ortho. Rel. Research*, 200, (Nov. 1985), pp. 50-53.

Dangberg, Grace, "Eliza Cook, M. D.," *Carson Valley Historical Sketches of Nevada's First Settlement*, (Carson Valley Hist. Soc., 1972).

Deshon, George D., "LTC George D. Deshon in His Own Words: The Career of a Medical Soldier 100 Years Ago," *Museum Notes*, Army Medical Department Center & School, Fort Sam Houston, Texas.

Duffy, John, "Medicine in the West: An Historical Overview," *J. West*, XXI, no. 3, (July 1982), pp. 5-14.

Evans, Richard J., "Epidemics and Revolution: Cholera in 19th-Century Europe," *Past & Present*, 120 (Aug. 1988), pp. 123-146.

Faust, Ernest Carroll, "Clinical and Public Health Aspects of Malaria in the United States from an Historical Perspective," *Amer. J. Tropical Med.*, 25 1945, pp. 185-201.

Fife, Austin E., "Pioneer Mormon Remedies," *West. Folklore*, 16 (3), 1957, pp. 153-162.

Furley, C.C., "Prophylactic Use of Cold Water in Parturition," *Pacific Med. Surg. J.*, 7 (June 1873) p. 183.

Giffen Helen S., "Camp Independence—An Owens Valley Outpost," *Quart., Hist. Soc. So. Cal.*, v. XXIV, (Dec. 1942), pp. 128-42.

Gross, Samuel D., "The Factors of Disease and Death After Injuries, Parturition, and Surgical Operations," *Public Health: Reports and Papers, II (1874-75)* pp. 400-414.

Gwyther, Surgeon George, "Scout to Black Canyon," *Overland Monthly*, 1st series, v. V (1870) pp. 221-531.

_____. "A Frontier Post and Country," *Overland Monthly*, 1st series, v. V (1870), p. 520-526.

_____. "An Indian Reservation," *Overland Monthly*, 1st series, v. X 1873, p. 123-134.

_____. "Pueblo Indians," *Overland Monthly*, March 1871.

Hardesty, Donald, "Historical Archaeology at Fort Churchill," *Nev. Hist. Soc. Quart.*, v. 24, no. 4, (Winter 1981), pp. 283-297.

Housley, Harold, "Notes and Documents: Elwood Decker and the CCC at Fort Churchill," *Nev. Hist. Soc. Quart.*, v. 38, no. 2, (Summer 1995).

Hume, Edgar Erskine, "Admission to the Medical Department of the Army Half a Century Ago: The Experience of Brigadier-General William Hemple Arthur," *Mili. Surg.*, 79 (1936), pp. 197-202.

The Inyo, (California), *Independent*, Mar. 3, 10, 17, and July 14, 1877.

Johnson, Norman K., "Taking a page from the Canny Comanche, Henry Sibley Devised a New Tent for the Western Frontier." *Wild West.* (Oct. 1991), p. 8.

Kampmeier, Rudolph, "Venereal Disease in the U.S. Army, 1775-1900." *Sexually Transmitted Disease*, 9 (Apr.-June 1982), pp. 100-103.

Kaufman, Howard H., "Treatment of Head Injuries in the American Civil War," *J. Neurosurg.*, 78 (May 1993), pp. 838-845.

Kober, George Martin, "The Progress and Tendency of Hygiene and Sanitary Science in the 19th Century," *Med. Record*, 59 (1901), pp. 898-906.

_____. "Report of a Case of Gunshot Wound of the Right Knee Joint and Right Hand." *Amer. J. Med. Sci.* New Series, 72 (1876), pp. 427-431.

Leland, Joy, ed., *Frederick West Lander: A Biograpical Sketch (1822-1862)*, Reno: Desert Research Inst. Pub., 1993.

Lorenz, Anthony J., "Scurvy in the Gold Rush," *J. Hist. Med. & Allied Sci.*, XII (1957).

Matthews, Surgeon Washington, "The Diary of," Ray H. Mattison, ed., *No. Dakota Hist.*, v. XXI, nos. 1 and 2 (Jan.-Apr., 1954).

McKeown, Thomas and R. G. Record, "Reasons for the Decline of Mortality in England and Wales during the 19th Century," *Population Studies*, 16 (1962-63), pp. 94-122.

"Medical School Directory of Graduates 1864-1921," *Univ. Calif. Bull.*, Third Series V, XV, no. 3, (1921).

Menzies, Richard, "Where the Steer and the Antelope Play," *Range Mag.* 1, no. 2, Fall/Winter 1992, pp. 32-36.

Morgan, James P., "The First Reported Case of Electrical Stimulation of the Human Brain," *J. Hist. Med. & Allied Sci.*, 37, no. 1, Jan. 1982, pp. 51-64.

Morrell, Joseph R., "Medicine of the Pioneer Period in Utah," *Utah Hist. Quart.*, XXIII (1955), pp. 127-144.

Munroe, Dot, The Diary of Dot Monroe—1886-1889, *J. Modoc Co. Hist. Soc.*, no. 10, 1988, pp. 13-60.

Olch, Peter D., "Medicine in the Indian-Fighting Army, 1866-1890." *J. West* XXI, no. 3 (July 1982) pp. 32-41.

Pond, William M., "The Mysterious Ending of Edward McGarry, *Periodical, J. Council Amer. Military Past*, v. XVII, no. 2, Apr. 1990.

Prendergast, H. L., "Quackery and the Quacked," *Nat. Quart. Rev.*, 1-2 (1860-1861), pp. 354-359.

Ramsey, Matthew, "The Politics of Professional Monopoly in 19th Century Medicine: The French Model and Its Rivals," Gerald Geison, ed., *Professions and the French State, 1700-1900.* (Philadelphia: Univ. Penn. Press, 1984), pp. 225-306.

Read, Georgia W., "Diseases, Drugs and Doctors on the Oregon-California Trail in the Gold-Rush Years," *Mo. Hist. Rev.*, XXXVIII (Apr. 1944), pp. 260-276.

Rocha, Guy Louis, "'Big Bill' Haywood and Humboldt County: The Making of a Revolutionary," *No. Cent. Nev. Hist. Soc. Quart.* VIII, Issue 2 & 3, pp. 3-27.

Ruhlen, Col. George, "Early Nevada Forts," *Nev. Hist. Soc. Quart.*, VII (1964).

San Francisco Morning Call, Feb. 6, 1891, and Apr. 28, 1892.

Shryock, Richard H., "A Medical Perspective on the Civil War," *Amer. Quart.*, 14 (1962), pp. 161-73.

Silver State (Nevada), 1886-87; May 19, 1875, 3;3; July 3, 1875, 3;1; Nov. 3, 1875, 3;1; and Dec. 23, 1875, 3;1.

Smith, Dale C., "Quinine and Fever: The Development of the Effective Dosage," *J. Hist. Med. & Allied Sci.*, 3, no. 3., July 1976, pp. 343-367.

Smith, Phillip Dodd, Jr., "The Sagebrush Soldiers: Nevada Volunteers in the Civil War," *Nev. Hist. Soc. Quart.*, 5, No. 3-4 (1987), pp. 3-87.

Sohn, Anton P., "19th-Century Academic Examinations for Physicians in the United States Army Medical Department," *West. J. Med.*, 160, no 5 (1994) pp. 472-474.

Virginia (Nevada), *Evening Bulletin*, Feb. 1864.

Virginia (Nevada), *Evening Chronicle*, Apr. 11, 1899.

Weir, James A., "The Army Doctor Looks at Indian Medicine," *Denver Westerners' Roundup*, 35, (Sept.-Oct. 1977), pp. 12-28.

Whitmore, Dr. William V., "Arizona's Pioneers in Medicine," *Ariz. Hist. Soc.*, Oct. 2, 1932.

Woyske, Margaret S., "Women and Mining in the Old West," *J. West*, XX (Apr. 1981), pp. 38-47.

UNPUBLISHED MANUSCRIPTS AND INTERVIEWS

Barry, Patricia A., Interview by the author, Fort Bidwell, California, May 15, 1994.

BeDunnah, Gary P., "A History of the Chinese in Nevada, 1855-1904: A Thesis," San Francisco, R & E Research Associates, 1973.

Chismore, George, "Journals," Bancroft Library, Univ. of Calif., Berkeley.

Corbusier, Fanny D., "Recollections of Her Life in the Army," Personal Diary.

"Fort Douglas Medical History," Fort Douglas Military Museum, Salt Lake City.

Halleck, "Letters sent from," Northeast Nevada Museum, Elko, Nevada.

Jones, Anne, "The Medical and Business Career of Dr. Charles Carroll Furley," Depart. of Hist., Municipal Univ. of Wichita, KS, May 4, 1953.

Kirkpatrick, Charles A., "Journal of 1849-1850," Bancroft Library, Univ. of Calif., Berkeley.

Kober, George Martin, Manuscript, MS 315, Hist. Med. Div., Nat. Lib. Med., Bethesda, Maryland.

Luckey, Eugene, Author's telephone interview, Burns, Oregon, May 17, 1994.

"Medical Directory of the Pacific Coast, 1880-1881," Cal. State Lib.

National Archives:

Record Group 92, Entry 225, "Correspondence file, Ft. Churchill," Quartermaster General.

Record Group 94, Entry 544, "Field Records of Hospitals."

Record Group 94, Entry 547, Book no. 69, "Medical History of Posts, Fort Cameron Beaver."

Record Group 94, Entry 547, Book no. 101, 104 and 106, "Medical History of Posts, Fort Bidwell."

Record Group 94, Entry 547, Book no. 126 and 224, "Medical History of Posts, Fort Harney."

Record Group 94, Entry 547, Book no. 135 and 234, "Medical History of Posts, Fort Independence."

Record Group 94, Entry 547, Book no. 327 and 328, "Medical History of Posts, Fort Warner."

Record Group 94, Entry 547, Book no. 374 and 376, "Medical History of Posts, Camp Halleck."

Record Group 94, Entry 547, Book no. 410 and 411, "Medical History of Posts, Camp McDermit."

Record Group 94, Entry 561, "Medical Officer Files."

Record Group 112, Entry 88, "Records of Medical Officers."

Record Group 112, Entry 92, Bidwell, Cameron, Churchill, Crittenden, Douglas, Halleck, Harney, Independence, McDermit, McGarry, Rawlins, Ruby, "Posts and Stations of Medical Officers."

M617, Rolls 112, 113, Fort Bidwell, California, "Returns from U.S. Military Posts 1800-1916."

M617, Roll 174, Fort Cameron (Beaver), Utah, "Returns from U.S. Military Posts 1800-1916."

M617, Roll 208, Fort Churchill, Nevada, "Returns from U.S. Military Posts 1800-1916."

M617, Roll 268, Fort Crittenden (Floyd), Utah, "Returns from U.S. Military Posts 1800-1916."

M617, Rolls 324-327, Fort Douglas, Utag, "Returns from U.S. Military Posts 1800-1916."

M617, Rolls 439, 440, Fort Halleck, Nevada, "Returns from U.S. Military Posts 1800-1916."

M617, Roll 454, Fort Harney (Steele), Oregon, "Returns from U.S. Military Posts 1800-1916."

M617, Roll 506, Fort Independence, California, "Returns from U.S. Military Posts 1800-1916."

M617, Roll 672, Camp McGarry, Nevada, "Returns from U.S. Military Posts 1800-1916."

M617, Roll 874, Camp Nye, Nevada, "Returns from U.S. Military Posts 1800-1916."

M617, Roll 1047, Camp Ruby, Nevada, "Returns from U.S. Military Posts 1800-1916."

M617, Roll 1273, Fort Three Forks of the Owyhee Winthrop, Idaho, "Returns from U.S. Military Posts."

M617, Roll 1352, Fort Warner, Oregon, "Returns from U.S. Military Posts 1800-1916."

M617, Roll 1447, Camp Winfield Scott, Nevada, "Returns from U.S. Military Posts 1800-1916."

M617, Roll 1535, Fort Rawlins, Utah, "Returns from U.S. Military Posts 1800-1916."

Saint Mary Louise Admission Records, Virginia City, Nevada.

S.G.O., "Autobiographical Sketches of Medical Officers," MS C44, Cit. No. 2933044R, Hist. Med. Div., Nat. Lib. Med., Bethesda, Maryland.

Wright, Earl, Interview by Edna Patterson, Elko, NV, July 29, 1958.

Index